W9-AYZ-018

THE SHREDDED CHEF

120 RECIPES FOR BUILDING MUSCLE, GETTING LEAN, AND STAYING HEALTHY

Michael Matthews

oculus

Copyright © 2013 by Oculus Publishers.

All rights reserved. This book or any portion thereof may not be reproduced or used in any manner whatsoever without the express written permission of the publisher except for the use of brief quotations in a book review. The scanning, uploading, and distribution of this book via the Internet or via any other means without the permission of the publisher is illegal and punishable by law.

Please purchase only authorized editions of this book and don't participate in or encourage electronic piracy of copyrighted materials.

If you would like to share this book with another person, please purchase an additional copy for each person you share it with, or ask them to buy their own copies. This was hard work for the author and he appreciates it.

This book is a general educational health-related information product and is intended for healthy adults, age 18 and over.

This book is solely for information and educational purposes and is not medical advice. Please consult a medical or health professional before you begin any exercise, nutrition, or supplementation program or if you have questions about your health.

There may be risks associated with participating in activities or using products mentioned in this book for people in poor health or with pre-existing physical or mental health conditions.

Because these risks exist, you should not use such products or participate in such activities if you are in poor health or have a pre-existing mental or physical health condition. If you choose to participate in these risks, you do so of your own free will and accord knowingly and voluntarily, assuming all risks associated with such activities.

Specific results mentioned in this book should be considered extraordinary and there are no "typical" results. As individuals differ, then results will differ.

ISBN-978-1-938895-08-1

Cover Designed by Damon Freeman

Photography by Emily Hillman

Typesetting by Kiersten Lief

Published by Oculus Publishers

www.oculuspublishers.com

Visit the author's website:

www.muscleforlife.com

ABOUT THE AUTHOR

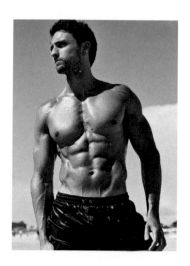

Hi,

I'm Mike and I've been training for nearly a decade now.

I believe that every person can achieve the body of his or her dreams, and I work hard to give everyone that chance by providing workable, proven advice grounded in science, not a desire to sell phony magazines, workout products, or supplements.

Through my work, I've helped thousands of people achieve their health and fitness goals, and I share everything I know in my books.

So if you're looking to get in shape and look great, then I think I can help you. I hope you enjoy my books and I'd love to hear from you at my site, www.muscleforlife.com.

Sincerely,

Mike

THE SHREDDED CHEF

When you wake up, your body is starved for nutrients. Feed it right! This section has breakfast recipes for getting big, for getting ripped, and it even includes some baking!

In this section, you'll find the following recipes:

Never be bored with a poultry dish again! This section has chicken and turkey recipes for getting big, for getting ripped, and it has 5 of my favorite marinades!

In this section, you'll find the following recipes:

It's hard to beat beef when it comes to building muscle, and in this section, you'll learn some of my favorite dishes!

This section has beef recipes for getting big and for getting ripped.

In this section, you'll find the following recipes:

Pork tenderloin is a great source of lean protein, and it can be prepared in many ways!

In this section, you'll find the following recipes:

Fish is one of the healthiest sources of protein you can eat and perfect for getting lean.

In this section, you'll find the following recipes:

Whole grains are a great source of slow-burning carbohydrates and fiber.

In this section, you'll find the following recipes:

Chicken Fettuccine with Mushrooms

Pasta Salad with Chicken

Beef Lasagna

Asparagus and Goat Cheese Pasta

Pork Tenderloin Stir-Fry

Delicious salads with tasty, low-calorie dressings are a great addition to every diet.

In this section, you'll find the following recipes:

Red Wine Vinaigrette Dressing

Balsamic Vinaigrette

Creamy White Vinegar Dressing

Steak and Sweet Potato Salad

Classic Cobb Salad

Spinach & Salmon Salad

Quick & Easy Protein Salad

Tropical Chicken Salad

Great side dishes are a perfect way to add some excitement and variety of taste to your meals.

In this section, you'll find the following recipes:

Green Beans Almondine

Baked Yellow Squash

Roasted Garlic Twice-Baked Potato

Sweet Potato Chips

PROTEIN SHAKES   201

Protein shakes are a great way to meet daily nutrition requirements, and are especially good for post-workout meals.

In this section, you'll find the following recipes:

PROTEIN BARS AND SNACKS   209

Learn how to make your own healthy protein bars using high-quality ingredients, plus a few other yummy snacks!

In this section, you'll find the following recipes:

Protein Pudding Bars

Strawberry Banana Protein Bars

No-Fat Tzatziki Sauce

Egg White Bites

Mean Green Salsa

Sizzling Salsa

Corn Tortilla Chips

Perfect Guacamole

Garlic Vegetable Dip

Everyone likes a tasty indulgence now and then, so I haven't forgotten the sweets.

In this section, you'll find the following recipes:

Protein Pudding

Peach Cobbler

Key Lime Pie

Protein Milkshake

Honey-Balsamic Strawberries

Chances are you'd like to use the recipes in this book to plan out your meals. This handy spreadsheet will help! In it you'll find a list of every recipe in the book along with their calories, protein, carbs, and fats!

BUILD MUSCLE AND LOSE FAT BY EATING TASTY, NUTRITIOUS FOOD

I used to hate cooking because I sucked at it.

Literally everything I made tasted horrible—and it took way too long.

To make things worse, I'm into weight lifting and had to eat a lot of that crappy food every week.

When I was eating to gain muscle, I couldn't really enjoy it because I didn't know how to make tasty meals that gave me enough calories and macronutrients (protein, carbs, and fats). I basically felt like a farm animal hitting the daily trough of chicken, eggs, oatmeal, brown rice, and potatoes.

When I was dieting to lose weight, well, I cringe when I think of the bland, plain chicken breasts and vegetables that I used to force down every day for months (I became quite a connoisseur of hot sauce, but eventually even that couldn't redeem the food). I would get excited over the banana I got to have with my afternoon shake. My buddies joked that I had the palate of a Rottweiler.

Finally, after years of desensitizing myself to food, I decided to figure out how to cook fast, healthy meals that tasted good and also met my nutritional needs. I wanted to look forward to hearty, nutritious meals when eating to gain muscle, and I wanted to enjoy some of what I got to eat while losing weight.

This book is a compilation of recipes that fit the bill. Every recipe in this book is designed to help you build lean muscle or lose fat while actually getting healthier (because who cares if you look great but feel like crap?). And they all TASTE GOOD.

So why buy this book?

Because following a diet, whether to get bigger or lose fat, is SO much more pleasurable when you can enjoy your meals. I think this book will become a good friend.

WHAT MAKES
THE SHREDDED CHEF
DIFFERENT?

As you probably know, you *must* eat properly to see good results from working out. You can grind away on the treadmill and pound weights until the cows come home and still see little to no results if you don't know how to support those activities with the right nutrition.

Muscles can't grow unless the body has the right nutrients to repair the damage caused by lifting weights. Eat too little, and you can not only fail to make gains, but you can actually lose muscle.

Your body can't lose fat unless you make it operate at just the right deficit of calories. Eat just a few hundred too many calories per day, and you'll find yourself stuck in the miserable rut of feeling like you're "on a diet" without losing any weight.

That being said, many diet plans out there exist in a vacuum. That is, they assume that eating conditions will always remain the same. They don't take into account the fact that most people can't stomach the same handful of food options every day, or that being severely restricted in one's diet can lead to all-out splurging, which then leads to the dreaded weight yo-yo.

What's needed is *balance*—a diet that allows for a variety of foods and that allows you to indulge now and again. It also has to be simple and practical so as to fit in with the craziness of our daily lives. And last but not least, it needs to enhance your overall health by incorporating healthy carbs and fats instead of the junk found in most people's fridges.

Well, that's what *The Shredded Chef* is all about. If you follow the advice given in this book, you'll not only find it easy to follow diets to gain muscle or lose fat, but you'll also be able to actually enjoy them.

As you'll see, most of the recipes are sorted into two categories: recipes for getting big and recipes for getting lean.

Recipes for getting big are going to be higher-calorie meals with a fair amount of carbs and fats, and they'll help you reach your daily calorie needs for building muscle.

Recipes for getting lean are lower-calorie meals with few carbs and fats, which is vital for dieting successfully.

You can, of course, eat any of the recipes whether you're trying to build muscle or lose weight. You simply have to ensure whatever you eat fits within your dietary plan.

So yes, this is a cookbook, but it's also going to teach you a bit about how to use these recipes to get bigger, leaner, and stronger...*and* healthier. And with 120 recipes, I think you'll get quite a lot of use out of this book.

HOW TO EAT RIGHT WITHOUT OBSESSING OVER EVERY CALORIE

I have good news.

You can look and feel great without breaking out a calculator every time you eat.

Getting proper nutrition is a precise science, but it doesn't have to be agonizing. In fact, I recommend a more laid-back approach. If you make planning or tracking meals too complicated, you'll have trouble sticking with it.

That being said, in order to lose fat, you must keep your body burning more energy than you're feeding it, and the energy potential of food is measured in calories. Eat too many calories—give your body more potential energy than it needs—and it has no incentive to burn fat.

In order to gain muscle, your body needs a surplus of energy to repair and rebuild itself (along with plenty of protein). Thus, you need to eat slightly more than your body burns to get bigger.

In this chapter I'm going to share some simple rules that you can follow to eat right. Just by following these rules, you'll find that you can lose or gain weight when you want to and that you'll feel healthy and vital.

1. MAKE SURE YOU EAT ENOUGH

A calorie is a measurement of the potential energy found in food, and your body burns quite a bit of energy every day. Everything from the beating of your heart to the digestion of your food requires energy, and your body has to get it from the food you eat.

Thus, it's important that you feed your body enough, and that's especially true when you work out. If you underfeed your body, don't be surprised if you don't have the energy to train hard or if you feel generally exhausted.

If you exercise at least three times per week, use the following formula to ensure you're feeding your body enough to repair itself.

- Eat 1 gram of protein per pound of body weight per day.

- Eat 1.5 grams of carbs per pound of body weight per day.

- Eat 1 gram of healthy fats per 4 pounds of body weight per day.

That's where you start. For a 130 lb woman, it would look like this:

- 130 grams of protein per day

- 195 grams of carbs per day

- 32 grams of fat per day

That's about 1,600 calories per day, which should work for making slow, steady muscle and strength gains without any fat added along the way (which really should be the goal of "maintenance"—not staying exactly the same).

If your priority is to gain muscle, then you need to add about 500 calories per day to your "maintenance" diet. The easiest way to do this is to bump up your carbs by about 50 grams per day, and your fats by about 30 grams per day.

If you're trying to lose fat, then you need to decrease your "maintenance" calories by about 20%. The easiest way to do this is to primarily reduce your carbs (don't drop your fats to less than 15-20% of your daily calories).

It's also important that you consume high-quality calories. Junk food calories, such as white bread, pastas, chips, juice and soda, will make you look and feel like crap, while good calories, such as fruits, vegetables, whole grains, and lean proteins, will keep you in tip-top shape.

2. EAT ENOUGH PROTEIN

If you work out, you need more protein than someone who doesn't work out. Why? Because exercise causes muscle damage.

With every rep you perform, you're causing "micro-tears" in your muscle fibers, and your body needs protein to fully repair this damage. The body doesn't just repair them to their previous state, however; it builds them bigger and stronger so it can better handle the stress of exercise.

So, in order to get the most out of your workouts, you need to eat enough protein. And that doesn't mean just eating a lot after working out. It means eating enough every day, which will require you to eat some with every meal you have (and as a general rule, eating .75 – 1 gram of protein per pound of body weight is a good target if you exercise regularly).

By doing this, you can ensure your body has the amino acids it needs to build muscle and repair tissue. If you fail to feed your body enough protein, it will fall behind in the muscle breakdown and repair cycle, and you can actually get smaller and weaker despite exercise.

There are two main sources of protein out there: whole food protein and supplement protein.

Whole food protein is, as you guessed, protein that comes from natural food sources, such as beef, chicken, fish, etc. The best forms of whole food protein are chicken, turkey, lean red meat, fish, eggs, and milk.

If you're vegetarian, your best options are eggs, low-fat cottage cheese (Organic Valley is my favorite brand), low-fat European style (Greek) yogurt (0% Fage is my favorite), tempeh, tofu, quinoa, almonds, rice, and beans.

While we're on the subject of vegetarianism, some people claim that you must carefully combine your proteins if you're vegetarian or vegan to ensure your body is getting "complete" proteins (all of the amino acids needed to build tissue). This theory and the faulty research it was based on was thoroughly debunked as a myth by the American

Dietetic Association, yet it still hangs around. While it's true that some sources of vegetable protein are lower in certain amino acids than other forms of protein, there is no scientific evidence to prove that they lack them altogether.

Protein supplements are powdered or liquid foods that contain protein from various sources, such as whey (a liquid remaining after milk has been curdled and strained in the process of making cheese), egg, and soy—the three most common sources of supplement protein. There are also great plant-based supplements out there that are a blend of high-quality protein sources such as quinoa, brown rice, peas, hemp, and fruit.

You don't NEED protein supplements to eat well, but it can be impractical for some to try to get all their protein from whole foods considering the fact that you will be eating protein 4 – 6 times per day.

Now, there are a few things you should know about eating protein. First is the subject of how much protein you can absorb in one sitting. Studies relating to this are very contradictory and disputed, mainly because it's a complex subject. Your genetics, metabolism, digestive tract health, lifestyle, and amount of lean mass are all important factors. But in the spirit of keeping things simple, here's what we know: you can eat and properly use a lot of protein in each meal. How much, exactly? Well, your body should have no trouble absorbing upwards of 100 grams in one sitting.

That said, there aren't any benefits of eating this way (I find gorging quite uncomfortable, actually), but it's good to know in case you miss a meal and need to make it up by loading protein into a later meal.

Another thing to know about protein is that different proteins digest at different speeds, and some are better utilized by the body than others. Beef protein, for example, is digested quickly, and 70 – 80% of what's eaten is utilized by the body (the exact number varies based on what study you read, but they all fall between 70 – 80%). Whey protein is also digested quickly and its "net protein utilization" (NPU) is in the low 90% range. Egg protein digests much slower than whey and beef, and its NPU also falls in the same range.

NPU and digestion speeds are important to know because you want to rely on high-NPU proteins to meet your daily protein requirement, and you want a quick-digesting protein for your post-workout meal, and a slow-digesting protein for your final meal before you go to bed (to help you get through the fasting that occurs during sleep).

I could give you charts and tables of the NPU rates of various proteins, but I'm going to keep it simple. In order to meet your daily protein requirements, here are your choices:

Whole Food Proteins

Lean meats (beef, pork, chicken, and turkey)

Fish

Eggs

Vegetarian sources noted above

Protein Supplements

Egg

Whey

Casein

In case you're wondering why I left soy protein off the list of recommended supplements, it's because it's just a bad protein source. To start, most soy protein supplements use genetically modified soybeans (which is a very dangerous trend encroaching further and further into the world of agriculture), and studies have shown that too much soy can increase estrogen levels and inhibit your body's testosterone production (due to a plant estrogen found in soybeans). Just stay away from it.

3. EAT HEALTHY FATS

Fats are the densest energy source available to your body. Each gram of fat contains over twice the calories of a gram of carbohydrate or protein. Healthy fats, such as those found in olive oil, avocados, flax seed oil, many nuts, and other foods, are actually an important component for overall good health. Fats help your body absorb the other nutrients that you give it; they nourish the nervous system, help maintain cell structures, regulate hormone levels, and more.

Saturated fats are a form of fat found mainly in animal products such as meat, dairy products, and egg yolks. Some plant foods, such as coconut oil, palm oil, and palm kernel oil, are also high in saturated fats. While it's commonly believed that eating saturated fat harms your health, the opposite is actually true. Recent studies have shown that including saturated fats in your diet can reduce your risk of heart disease.

Trans fats are scientifically modified saturated fats that have been engineered to give foods longer shelf lives. Many cheap, packaged foods are full of trans fats (such as run-of-the-mill popcorn, yogurt, and peanut butter) as are many frozen foods (such as frozen pizza, packaged pastries, cakes, etc.). And fried foods are often fried in trans fats. These fats are bad news, and eating too much of them can lead to all kinds of diseases and complications. They have no nutritional value for the body and thus should be avoided altogether.

Most people eat more fat than is necessary, thus adding lots of unnecessary calories to their daily intake. Getting enough healthy fats every day is pretty simple. Here's how it works:

- Keep your intake of saturated fats relatively low (below 10% of your total calories). Saturated fat is found in foods like meat, dairy products, eggs, coconut oil, bacon fat, and lard. If a fat is solid at room temperature, it's a saturated fat.

- Completely avoid trans fats. Trans fats are found in processed foods such as cookies, cakes, fries, and doughnuts. Any food that contains "hydrogenated oil" or "partially hydrogenated oil" likely contains trans fats, so just don't eat it. (Sure, having a cheat here and there that contains trans fats won't harm anything, but you definitely don't want to eat them regularly.)

- Get at least half of your daily fat from unsaturated fats such as olive oil, nuts, peanut oil, avocados, flax seed oil, safflower oil, or sesame oil. If a fat is liquid at room temperature, it's an unsaturated fat.

By simply sticking to the recipes in this book, you'll avoid unhealthy fats and include healthy fats without even trying.

4. EAT GOOD CARBS

The carbohydrate is probably the most misunderstood, maligned, and feared macro-nutrient. Thanks to the scores of bogus diet plans and suggestions out there, many people equate eating carbs with getting fat. While eating TOO MANY carbs can make you fat (just as eating too much protein or fat can), carbs are hardly your enemy. They play an essential role in not only muscle growth but in overall body function.

Regardless of what type of carbohydrate you eat—broccoli or apple pie—the body breaks it down into two substances: glucose and glycogen. Glucose is commonly referred to as "blood sugar," and it's an energy source used by your cells to do the many things they do. Glycogen is a substance stored in the liver and muscles that can be easily converted to glucose for immediate energy. When you lift weights intensely, your muscles burn up their glycogen stores to cope with the overload.

Now, why is broccoli good for you but apple pie isn't? Because your body reacts very differently to broccoli than to apple pie. You've probably heard the terms "simple" and "complex" carbs before and wondered what they meant. You might have also heard of the glycemic index and wondered what it was all about.

These things are actually pretty simple. The glycemic index is a numeric system of ranking how quickly carbohydrates are converted into glucose in the body. Carbs are ranked on a scale of 0 to 100 depending how they affect blood sugar levels once eaten. A GI rating of 55 and under is considered "low GI," 56 to 69 is medium, and 70 and above is high on the index. A "simple" carb is one that converts very quickly (is high on the glycemic index), such as table sugar, honey, and watermelon, while a "complex" carb is one that converts slowly (is low on the glycemic index), such as broccoli, apple, and whole-grain bread.

It's very important to know where the carbs you eat fall on the index, because studies have linked regular consumption of high-GI carbs to increased risk for heart disease, diabetes, and obesity.

The amount of carbohydrates that you should eat every day depends on what you're trying to accomplish. Building muscle requires that you eat a substantial amount of carbs, while dieting to lose weight requires that you reduce carbs.

Regardless of how many carbs you need to eat per day, there's a simple rule to follow regarding high-, medium- and low-glycemic carbs.

Eat carbs in the medium–high range of the glycemic index (60 – 90 is a good rule of thumb) about 30 minutes before you exercise, and again within 30 minutes of finishing your workout.

The reason you want some carbs before training is that you need the energy for your training. The reason you want them after is that your muscles' glycogen stores are heavily depleted, and by replacing glycogen quickly, you actually help your body maintain an anabolic state and not lose muscle tissue.

My favorite pre- and post-workout carbs are bananas and rice milk, but other good choices are baked potato, instant oatmeal, and fruits that are above 60 on the glycemic index, such as cantaloupe, pineapple, watermelon, dates, apricots, and figs. Some people recommend eating foods high in table sugar (sucrose) after working out because it's high on the GI, but I stay away from processed sugar as much as possible.

All other carbs you eat should be in the middle or at the low end of the glycemic index (60 and below is a good rule of thumb). It really is that simple. If you follow this rule, you'll avoid many problems that others suffer from due to the energy highs and lows that come with eating high-GI carbs that burn the body out.

Below is a list of common snack foods with corresponding average GI scores. The GI scores vary a bit from brand to brand, but not by much. Generally speaking, it's best to stay away from these types of carbs.

(The following information is sourced from the University of Sydney, the University of Harvard, and Livestrong.com.)

FOOD	GI
White bread bagel	72
Corn chips	63
Pretzels	83
Candy bar	62 – 78
Wheat or corn cracker	67 – 87
Rye cracker	64
Rice cake	78
Popcorn	72
White rice	64
Pizza	80
Raisins	64
Whole wheat bread	71
White bread	70
Baguette	95
English muffin (white bread)	77

Baked potato	85
Muesli	66

So, forget stuff like sugar, white bread, processed, low-quality whole wheat bread, bagels, junk cereals, muffins, white pasta, crackers, waffles, rice cakes, corn flakes, and white rice. I wouldn't even recommend eating these things often as pre- or post-workout carbs because they're just not good for your body.

Even certain fruits, such as watermelon and dates, are bad snack foods because of where they fall on the glycemic index. If you're unsure about a carb you like, look it up to see where it falls on the glycemic index. If it's above 60, just leave it out of your meals that aren't immediately before or after working out.

5. EAT YOUR FRUITS AND VEGGIES

Your body requires many different things to function optimally. It can't look and feel great on protein and carbs alone. You need calcium to ensure your muscles can contract and relax properly. You need fiber to help move food through the digestive tract. You need iron to carry oxygen to your cells and create energy.

There are many other "little helpers" that your body needs to perform its many physiological processes, and fruits and vegetables contain many vital nutrients that you can't get from vitamin supplements. By eating 3 – 5 servings of both fruits and vegetables per day, you enjoy the many benefits that these nutrients give to your body, such as lowering your risk of cancer, heart disease, diabetes, and many other diseases.

This isn't hard to do, either. A medium-sized piece of fruit is one serving, as is half a cup of berries. A cup of greens is a serving of vegetables, as is half a cup of other vegetables.

Fruit *juices*, however, are another story. While they may seem like an easy way to get in your daily fruits, they are actually not much more than tasty sugar water. Not only do most fruit juices have sugar added, but the juice has also been separated from the fruit's fibrous pulp, which slows down the metabolism of the sugars. Without that, the juice becomes a very high-glycemic drink. You're better off drinking water and eating whole fruit.

The exception to this is creating juice using a juicer or blender to grind up the entire piece of fruit, removing nothing. This, of course, is no different than chewing up the fruit in your mouth.

Fruits widely recognized as the healthiest are apples, bananas, blueberries, oranges, grapefruit, strawberries, and pineapples.

Vegetables often recommended as the healthiest are asparagus, broccoli, spinach, sweet potatoes, tomatoes, carrots, onions, and eggplant.

6. PLAN AND PROPORTION YOUR MEALS PROPERLY

Many people's meal plans are engineered for getting fat. They skip breakfast, eat a junk food lunch, come home famished, have a big dinner with some dessert, and then have a snack like chips or popcorn while watching TV at night.

A much better strategy is to eat smaller meals every 3 – 4 hours, and include protein with each (as this fills you up and makes you feel satisfied).

Much of your daily carbohydrates should come before and after training, when your body needs them most. I eat about 10 – 15% of my daily carbs before training, and about 30 – 40% after, in my post-workout meal.

It's also important when dieting to lose weight to not eat carbs within several hours of going to bed. This advice has been kicking around the health and fitness world for quite some time, but usually with the wrong explanation.

There's no scientific evidence that eating carbs at night or before bed will lead to gaining fat, but it can *hinder* fat loss. How?

The insulin created by the body to process and absorb carbs eaten stops the use of fat as an energy source. Your body naturally burns the most fat while sleeping, and so going to sleep with elevated insulin levels interferes with fat loss.

Related to this is the fact that studies have indicated that the production and processing of insulin interferes with the production and processing of growth hormone, which has powerful fat-burning properties. Your body naturally produces much of its growth hormone while sleeping, so again, if your body is flushed with insulin when you go to sleep, your growth hormone production may suffer, which in turn may rob you of its fat-burning and muscle-building benefits.

So, as a general rule, when you're dieting to lose weight, don't eat any carbs within 4 – 5 hours of bedtime. You should only consume lean proteins after dinner. I follow this rule when bulking too, not because

I'm worried about fat burning (you don't burn fat when bulking), but because I don't want to stunt my growth hormone production.

You can spread your fats throughout the day. I like to start my day with 1 – 2 tablespoons of a 3-6-9 blend (a combination of essential fatty acids, which are fats vital for the proper function of every cell, tissue, gland, and organ in your body), but you don't have to get one if you don't want to. You can simply stick to the sources of healthy fat given earlier.

7. DRINK A LOT OF WATER

The human body is about 60% water in adult males and about 70% in adult females. Muscles are about 70% water. That alone tells you how important staying hydrated is to maintaining good health and proper body function. Your body's ability to digest, transport, and absorb nutrients from food is dependent upon proper fluid intake. Water helps prevent injuries in the gym by cushioning joints and other soft-tissue areas. When your body is dehydrated, literally every physiological process is negatively affected.

I really can't stress enough the importance of drinking clean, pure water. It has zero calories, so it will never cause you to gain weight regardless of how much you drink. (You can actually harm your body by drinking too much water, but this would require that you drink several gallons per day.)

The Institute of Medicine reported in 2004 that women should consume about 91 ounces of water—or three-quarters of a gallon— per day, and men should consume about 125 ounces per day (a gallon is 128 ounces).

Now, keep in mind that those numbers include the water found in food. The average person gets about 80% of their water from drinking it and other beverages, and about 20% from the food they eat.

I've been drinking 1 – 2 gallons of water per day for years now, which is more than the IOM baseline recommendation, but I sweat a fair amount due to exercise and I live in Florida, which surely makes my needs higher. I fill a one-gallon jug at the start of my day and simply make sure that I finish it by dinner time. By the time I go to bed, I'll have drank a few more glasses.

Make sure the water you drink is filtered, purified water and not tap water. There's a big difference between drinking clean, alkaline water that your body can fully utilize and drinking polluted, acidic junk from the tap or bottle (which is the case with certain brands such as Dasani and Aquafina).

8. CUT BACK ON THE SODIUM

The average American's diet is so over-saturated with sodium it makes my head spin.

The Institute of Medicine recommends 1,500 milligrams of sodium per day as the adequate intake level for most adults. According to the CDC, the average American aged 2 and up eats *3,436 milligrams* of sodium per day.

Too much sodium in the body causes water retention (which gives you that puffy, soft look) and it can lead to high blood pressure and heart disease.

Frozen and canned foods are full of sodium, as are cured meats like bacon and sausage (one slice of bacon contains *1,000 milligrams* of sodium!).

Whenever possible, I chose low- or no-sodium ingredients for the recipes in this book. When you need to add salt, I recommend sea salt or Himalayan rock salt (sounds like fancy BS, but it's actually great stuff) because it has many naturally occurring minerals, whereas run-of-the-mill table salt has been "chemically cleaned" to remove "impurities," which includes these vital elements.

9. CHEAT CORRECTLY

Many people struggling with diets talk about "cheat days." The idea is that if you're good during the week, you can go buck wild on the weekends and somehow not gain fat. Well, unless you have a very fast metabolism, that's not how it works. If you follow a strict diet and exercise, you can expect to lose 1 – 2 pounds per week. If you get too crazy, you can gain it right back over a weekend.

So don't think cheat DAYS, think cheat MEALS—meals where you eat more or less anything you want (and all other meals of the week follow your meal plan). When done once or twice per week, a cheat meal is not only satisfying, but it can actually help you lose fat.

How?

Well, first there's the psychological boost, which keeps you happy and motivated, which ultimately makes sticking to your diet easier.

But there's also a physiological boost.

Studies on overfeeding (the scientific term for binging on food) show that doing so can boost your metabolic rate by anywhere from 3 – 10%. While this sounds good, it actually doesn't mean much when you consider that you would need to eat anywhere from a few hundred to a few thousand extra calories in a day to achieve this effect.

More important are the effects cheating has on a hormone called leptin, which regulates hunger, your metabolic rate, appetite, motivation, and libido, as well as serving other functions in your body.

When you're in a caloric deficit and lose body fat, your leptin levels drop. This, in turn, causes your metabolism to slow down, your appetite to increase, your motivation to wane, and your mood to sour.

On the other hand, when you give your body more energy (calories) than it needs, leptin levels are boosted, which can then have positive effects on fat oxidation, thyroid activity, mood, and even testosterone levels.

So if it's a leptin boost that you really want, how do you best achieve it?

Eating carbohydrates is the most effective way. Second to that is eating protein (high-protein meals also raise your metabolic rate). Dietary fats aren't very effective at increasing leptin levels, and alcohol actually inhibits it.

So, if your weight is stuck and you're irritable and demotivated, a nice kick of leptin might be all you need to get the scales moving again.

Have a nice cheat meal full of protein and carbs, and feel good about it.

(I would recommend, however, that you don't go too overboard with your cheat meals—don't eat 2,000 calories of junk food and desserts and think it won't do anything.)

How many cheat meals you should eat per week depends on what you're trying to accomplish.

When you're eating to stay lean and gain muscle slowly, two cheat meals per week is totally fine. When you're dieting to lose weight, you can have one cheat meal per week.

THE BOTTOM LINE

You may find this chapter a bit hard to swallow (no pun intended). Some people have a really hard time giving up their unhealthy eating habits (sugar and junk food can be pretty addictive). That being said, consider the following benefits of following the advice in this chapter:

1. If this is a completely new way of eating for you, I *guarantee* you'll feel better than you have in a *long* time. You won't have energy highs and lows. You won't feel lethargic. You won't have that mental fogginess that comes with being stuffed full of unhealthy food every day.

2. You will appreciate "bad" food so much more when you only have it once or twice per week. You'd be surprised how much better a dessert tastes when you haven't had one in a week. (You may also be surprised that junk food that you loved in the past no longer tastes good.)

3. You will actually come to enjoy healthy foods. I *promise*. Even if they don't taste good to you at first, just groove in the routine, and soon you'll crave brown rice and fruit instead of doughnuts and bread. Your body will adapt.

This chapter teaches you all there really is to eating properly so you can build muscle or lose weight on demand, all while staying healthy.

LET'S GET COOKING

Getting lean, while still feeding your muscles and body what they need, can be tough. That's why I wrote this book, and I'm confident that you'll be able to find the right recipes to fit your needs.

Nothing in this book is fancy or hard to make, yet many of the recipes are quite delicious. I'm sure that you'll find some new staples for your diet in this book.

For most of these recipes all you'll need is a couple pots and pans, and maybe a blender. The instructions are easy to follow, the prep times are minimal, and the ingredients are easy to find. Cooking doesn't get much simpler than this.

I recommend that you pick out a week's worth of recipes and then go shopping for the ingredients. Many of the recipes use the same ingredients, which will save you money and time.

So, let's get started!

BREAKFAST

For many years now, a staple in weight-loss plans and maintenance advice has been to make sure you eat a nice, big breakfast every day.

This is backed by observational research in which eating breakfast is associated with lower body weight in large populations, but it perfectly illustrates how bad advice can become so prevalent in this industry.

Observational research, which can't establish causation, suggests that something may be the case (skipping breakfast seems to be negatively associated with body weight), but indicates that more rigorous research is needed to see if there truly is a connection and why.

The media, however, jumps on such studies as cold, hard proof and starts running stories with headlines announcing "breakthrough" discoveries. Big health and fitness magazines and websites pick up on those stories for new content, trainers and gymgoers read it and spread it, and on it goes.

The side of the breakfast story you're not told is that research has shown that people who skip breakfast are more likely to eat junk food and tend to eat more in general. It wasn't the breakfast skipping that was causing the problem; it was the candy, soda, and excess calories. Breakfast eaters merely tend to maintain better overall dietary habits—no big surprise that they tend to be thinner as well.

So, eat breakfast if you like it (I do), especially if you find yourself very hungry when you wake up. But don't be afraid to delay it a couple of hours or skip it altogether and eat your first meal at lunch if that works better for you. (If you would like to know more about why fasting like this doesn't get in the way of muscle building or weight loss, and why it's actually healthy for you, read my book Muscle Myths.)

If you're pressed for time in the mornings, you can make some of the recipes in this section in advance and just keep them in the fridge. Or you can make quick meals like oatmeal or egg scrambles. And if you have a little time, and so desire, treat yourself to something like pancakes (one of my favorite cheat foods!).

BREAKFAST RECIPES FOR GETTING BIG

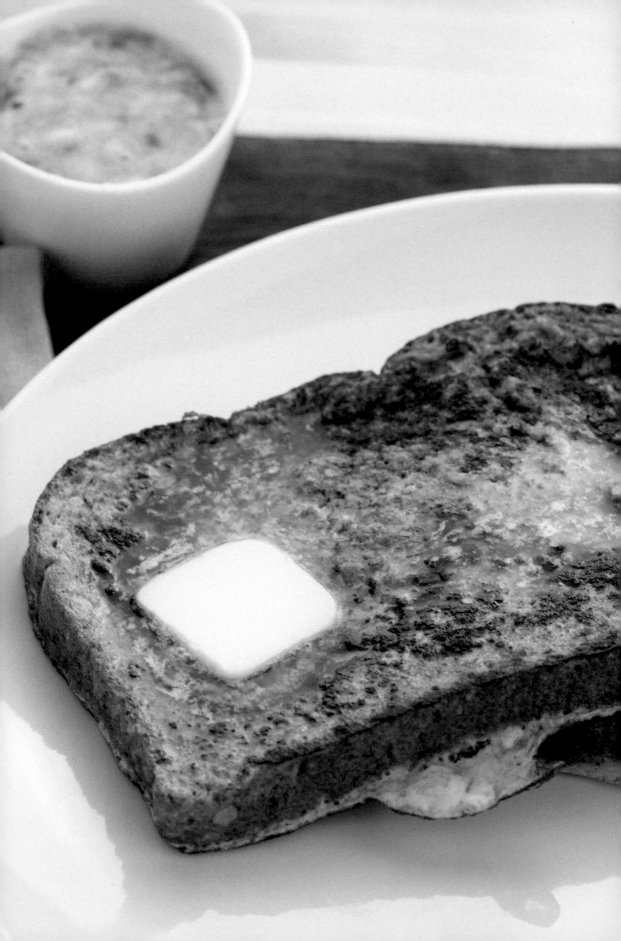

FRENCH MUSCLE TOAST

1/2 cup skim milk

2 large eggs

2 egg whites

2 scoops vanilla whey protein powder

1/2 teaspoon ground cinnamon

4 slices whole grain bread

FOR THE TOPPING:

1 banana, mashed

1 tablespoon strawberry preserves

1 tablespoon water

Servings	2 (2 pieces per serving)
Prep Time	5 mins
Cooking Time	5 – 10 mins

PER SERVING

Calories	445
Protein	44 grams
Carbohydrates	50 grams
Fat	9 grams

> Mix the skim milk, eggs, and egg whites together in a bowl. Then mix in the protein powder and cinnamon and beat until completely mixed.

> Soak a slice of bread in the mixture until soggy (I like to let it sit for 30 seconds or so).

> Coat a pan with cooking spray and heat on medium-high heat.

> Put one or two slices of bread into the pan and cook for 2 minutes or until golden brown. Then flip the slices and cook the other side for another 1 – 2 minutes or until fully cooked. The bread should no longer be soggy but firm instead.

> While cooking the bread, mix up the fruit and water in a bowl. Top off each slice of bread with a dollop.

Servings	2 (2 oatcakes per serving)
Prep Time	5 mins
Cooking Time	10 mins
PER SERVING	
Calories	351
Protein	31 grams
Carbohydrates	45 grams
Fat	6 grams

HIGH PROTEIN BANANA OATCAKES

1 cup old-fashioned oats

6 egg whites

1 ripe banana

1 cup low-fat cottage cheese

1/2 teaspoon ground cinnamon

1 teaspoon stevia or other sugar alternative

> Blend everything together until it's a smooth batter.

> Coat a pan with cooking spray and wipe away the excess with a paper towel. Save this for wiping the pan after cooking each pancake. Heat the pan on medium-low heat.

> Spoon about 1/2 cup of batter into the pan and cook for 1 – 2 minutes or until golden brown. Flip the pancake and cook for 30 seconds to 1 minute or until golden brown and firm. Put the pancake on a plate and wipe the pan with the paper towel.

> Repeat step 3 with the rest of the batter.

APPLE CINNAMON OATMEAL

Servings	4
Prep Time	5 mins
Cooking Time	2 – 3 mins
PER SERVING	
Calories	263
Protein	29 grams
Carbohydrates	30 grams
Fat	3 grams

1 1/2 cups quick cooking oats

1/3 cup nonfat dry milk powder (optional)

1/4 cup dried apples, diced

4 scoops chocolate whey protein powder

1 tablespoon brown sugar

1 tablespoon stevia or other sugar alternative

3/4 teaspoon ground cinnamon

1/4 teaspoon salt

1/8 teaspoon ground cloves

1/2 cup water (per serving)

> Mix all of the ingredients except the water in a large airtight container and store, good for up to 6 months.

> To prepare the oatmeal: Shake the container well to ensure the ingredients are well mixed. In a saucepan, bring 1/2 cup of water to a boil. Measure out and stir in 1/2 cup of the mixture, cook and stir for 1 minute over medium heat. Remove from the heat and cover, let sit for 1 minute or longer depending on desired consistency.

QUICK AND EASY PEANUT BUTTER OATMEAL

Servings	1
Prep Time	2 – 3 mins
Cooking Time	5 – 7 mins

PER SERVING

Calories	423
Protein	41 grams
Carbohydrates	35 grams
Fat	14 grams

1/2 cup old-fashioned oats

1/4 teaspoon salt

2 teaspoons ground flax seed

2 egg whites

2/3 cup water

1 tablespoon peanut butter

ground cinnamon, to taste

1 scoop chocolate whey protein powder

> Place oats in a deep microwave safe bowl. Stir in the salt and flaxseed. In a separate bowl, whisk together the egg whites and water, then pour over the oatmeal and stir gently until just combined.

> Microwave on medium for 4 – 6 minutes.

> Remove from microwave and stir in the peanut butter, cinnamon, and protein powder.

BAKED RAISIN OATMEAL

Servings	1
Prep Time	3 – 4 mins
Cooking Time	35 – 40 mins

PER SERVING

Calories	399
Protein	38 grams
Carbohydrates	42 grams
Fat	8 grams

1 teaspoon vegetable oil

1/2 teaspoon stevia or other sugar alternative

2 egg whites

2 tablespoons skim milk

1/8 teaspoon salt

1/4 teaspoon baking powder

1/2 cup quick cooking oats

1 scoop chocolate or vanilla whey protein powder

1 tablespoon raisins

1/2 teaspoon brown sugar

1/8 teaspoon ground cinnamon

> In a large mixing bowl, beat together the oil and stevia, slowly mix in the egg whites, skim milk, salt, baking powder, oats, protein powder, and raisins. Top with the brown sugar and cinnamon and place in refrigerator overnight.

> Heat the oven to 350°F, bake until firm, around 35 minutes.

SWEET POTATO PROTEIN PANCAKES

1 medium-sized sweet potato

1/2 cup old-fashioned oats

1 large egg

4 egg whites

1/2 teaspoon vanilla extract

1/2 teaspoon ground cinnamon

1/4 cup fat-free plain yogurt

Servings	1 (2 pancakes per serving)
Prep Time	10 mins
Cooking Time	5 mins

PER SERVING

Calories	358
Protein	24 grams
Carbohydrates	59 grams
Fat	3 grams

> Puncture the sweet potato several times with a fork. Wrap it in a paper towel and microwave it for 5 minutes on high. Run it under cool water and then remove the skin with a knife.

> Blend the oats until they are a powder and dump into a bowl. Blend the sweet potato until smooth and place it into the bowl with the oats. Stir in the egg, egg whites, vanilla extract, cinnamon, and yogurt. Mix well until it forms a smooth batter.

> Coat a pan with cooking spray and wipe away the excess with a paper towel. Save this for wiping the pan after cooking each pancake. Heat the pan on medium-low heat.

> Spoon about 1/2 cup of batter into the pan and cook for 1 – 2 minutes or until golden brown. Flip the pancake and cook for 30 seconds to 1 minute or until golden brown and firm. Put the pancake on a plate and wipe the pan with the paper towel.

> Repeat step 4 with the rest of the batter.

TURKEY BACON & VEGGIE OMELET

Servings	1
Prep Time	5 – 10 mins
Cooking Time	5 – 6 mins

PER SERVING

Calories	283
Protein	35 grams
Carbohydrates	8 grams
Fat	12 grams

1/2 cup fresh mushrooms, sliced

3 spears asparagus, cut into 2-inch pieces

1/3 cup scallions, chopped

5 egg whites

1 large egg

2 slices turkey bacon, cooked and cut into small slices

1 tablespoon low-fat Parmesan cheese, shredded

> Place a large skillet over medium heat, lightly coat in oil and, once hot, add the mushrooms, asparagus, and scallions. Cook, stirring occasionally until the asparagus is fairly soft, about 4 minutes.

> Whisk the eggs and pour over the vegetables, reduce heat to medium-low.

> While the omelet cooks, lift the edge to allow all of the uncooked egg to flow underneath. Once most of the egg is cooked, add the turkey bacon and cheese on top and let melt to desired consistency, fold the omelet in half and remove from heat.

SWEET POTATO & SAUSAGE FRITTATA

Servings	1
Prep Time	5 mins
Cooking Time	15 – 20 mins
PER SERVING	
Calories	425
Protein	43 grams
Carbohydrates	29 grams
Fat	17 grams

1 medium-sized sweet potato, cut into small cubes

1 link breakfast turkey sausage, chopped

1 egg

6 egg whites

1/4 cup low-fat cheddar cheese, shredded

salt and ground black pepper, to taste

1/8 cup tomato, chopped and seeded

1/8 cup scallions, thinly sliced

> Preheat the oven to 350°F.

> Coat a medium-sized oven-proof pan in cooking spray and place over medium heat. Put the potatoes in the pan and cover them for about 5 minutes. Add the sausage and cover, cook for another 4 – 5 minutes, stirring occasionally (you want to cook the sweet potatoes until slightly tender).

> Beat the eggs, cheese, salt, and pepper in a large mixing bowl with a whisk.

> Pour the egg mixture over the sweet potato and sausage and cook for about 5 – 6 minutes, or until the eggs are golden brown on the bottom.

> Transfer the pan to the oven for about 5 minutes, or until top is golden brown. Top with the tomatoes and scallions.

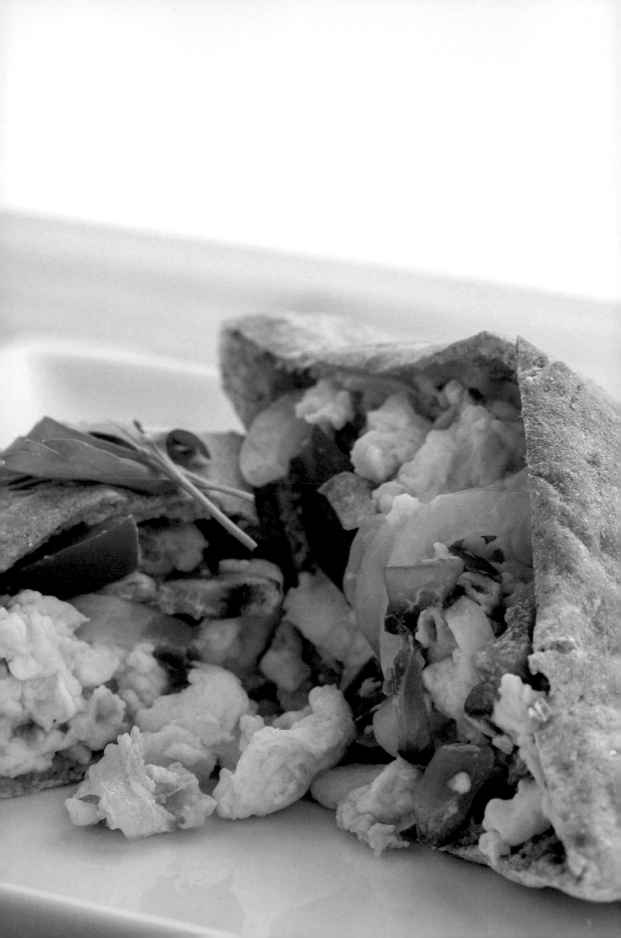

BREAKFAST PITA WRAP

Servings	1
Prep Time	5 mins
Cooking Time	8 – 10 mins

PER SERVING

Calories	452
Protein	31 grams
Carbohydrates	49 grams
Fat	20 grams

4 white mushrooms, sliced

1 tablespoon onion, chopped

1 tablespoon red bell pepper, chopped

pinch of ground black pepper

1 large egg

3 egg whites

1/2 small tomato, seeded and chopped

3 tablespoons skim milk

1 whole grain pita (choose the brand with the lowest fat and sodium), halved and toasted

1/2 avocado, sliced

> Coat a pan with cooking spray and cook the mushrooms, onion, and bell pepper on medium heat. Cook for 3 – 4 minutes. Add black pepper.

> Mix the egg, egg whites, tomato, and skim milk in a bowl and beat until frothy.

> Pour the egg mixture into the pan and cook for 3 – 4 minutes, stirring until firm.

> Fill each pita half with half of the egg mixture and half the avocado.

BREAKFAST RECIPES FOR GETTING LEAN

LEAN AND MEAN ZUCCHINI HASH

2 large eggs

1 cup zucchini, grated

1/4 cup onion, diced

1/4 teaspoon garlic powder

1/4 teaspoon onion powder

salt and ground black pepper, to taste

Servings	1
Prep Time	5 mins
Cooking Time	10 mins
PER SERVING	
Calories	202
Protein	15 grams
Carbohydrates	11 grams
Fat	11 grams

> Mix all the ingredients together in a bowl.

> Heat a pan on high and then lower to medium heat.

> Spray some cooking spray into the pan and spoon the mixture into it. Cook about 5 minutes and flip. Cook another 5 minutes.

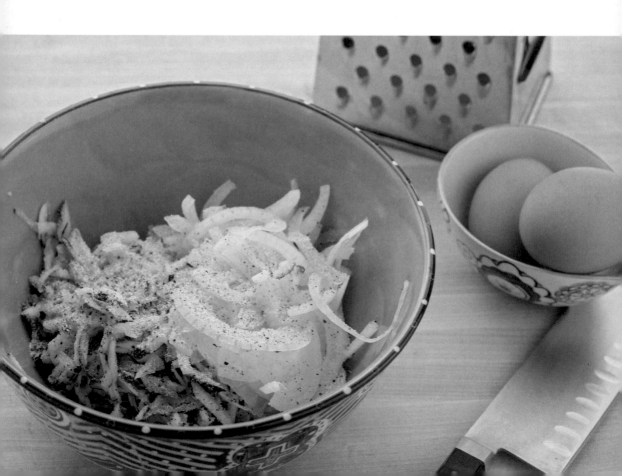

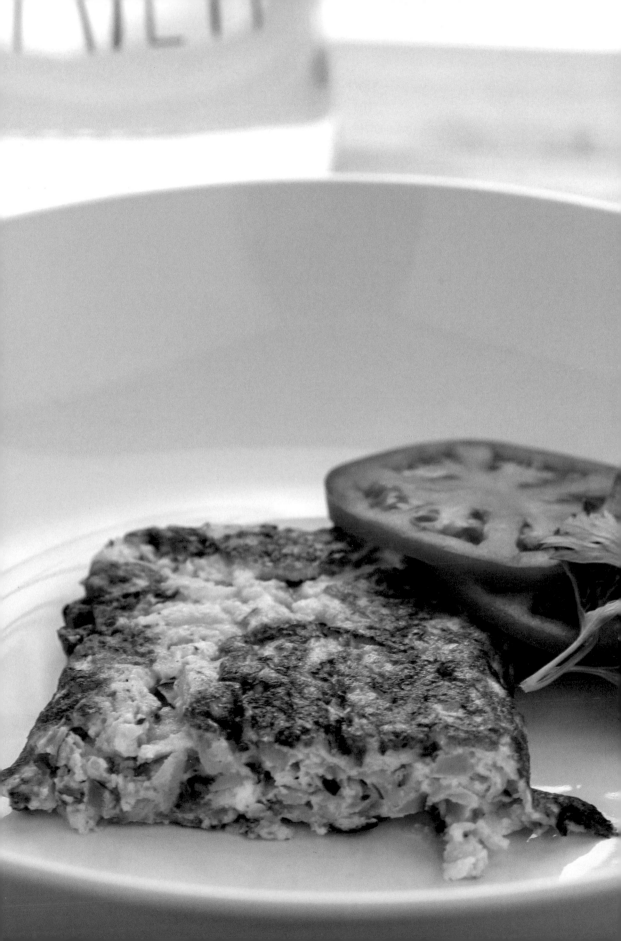

SIMPLE SPINACH SCRAMBLE

Servings	1
Prep Time	2 – 3 mins
Cooking Time	5 mins
PER SERVING	
Calories	275
Protein	36 grams
Carbohydrates	9 grams
Fat	10 grams

1 cup spinach (fresh or frozen)

1/4 cup onion, chopped

1/4 cup red bell pepper, chopped

6 egg whites

2 large eggs

salt and ground black pepper, to taste

> Clean the spinach off and throw it into a pan while still wet. Cook on medium heat and season with salt and pepper.

> Once the spinach is wilted, add the onion and bell pepper and cook until the onions are translucent and the pepper chunks are soft.

> Add the eggs and scramble until cooked. Top with salt and pepper.

ZUCCHINI FRITTATA

Servings	1
Prep Time	5 mins
Cooking Time	10 – 12 mins
PER SERVING	
Calories	214
Protein	31 grams
Carbohydrates	8 grams
Fat	7 grams

1/4 cup onion, chopped

1/2 cup zucchini, shredded

6 egg whites

1 large egg

salt and ground black pepper, to taste

1 tablespoon low-fat cheddar cheese, shredded

> Preheat the oven to 350°F.

> Coat an 8-inch oven-proof skillet in cooking spray and place over medium heat. Add the onion and zucchini and sauté for 2 – 3 minutes.

> In a large mixing bowl, whisk together the eggs. Pour over the top of vegetables, sprinkle with salt and pepper. Cook until almost set, about 6 – 7 minutes. Sprinkle the cheese on top and transfer to the oven. Bake for 4 – 5 minutes or until the cheese is melted.

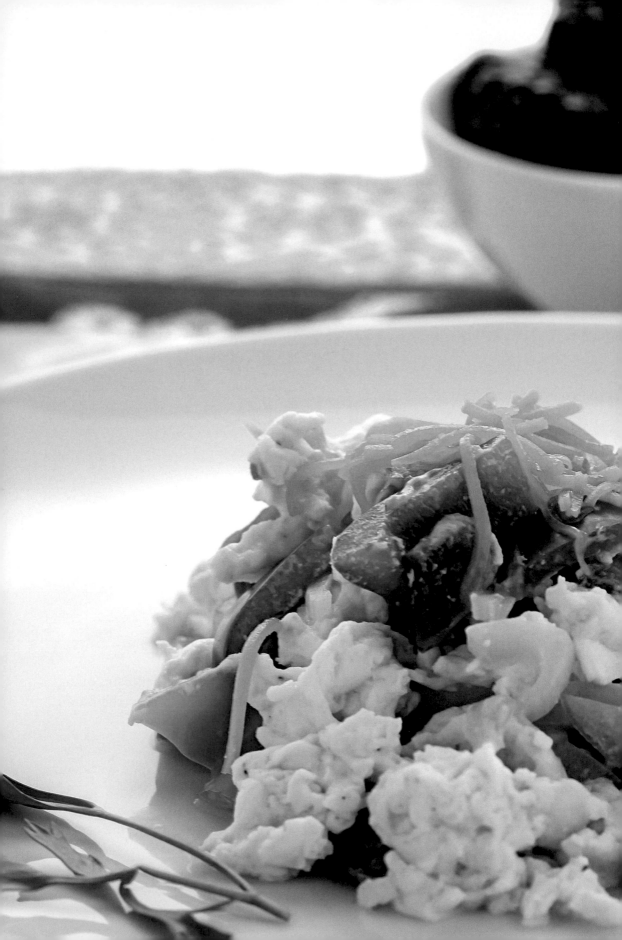

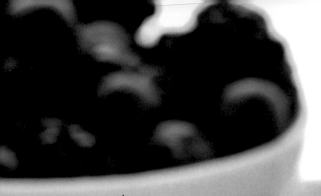

Servings	1
Prep Time	5 mins
Cooking Time	5 mins
PER SERVING	
Calories	235
Protein	33 grams
Carbohydrates	11 grams
Fat	8 grams

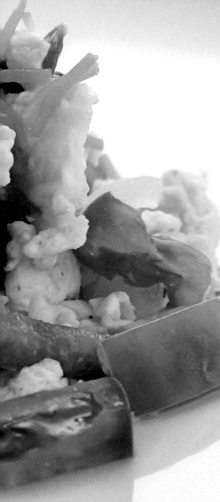

VEGGIE EGG & CHEESE SCRAMBLE

1/4 cup mushrooms, chopped

1/4 cup green bell peppers, chopped

1/4 cup onions, chopped

6 egg whites

1 large egg

2 tablespoons skim milk

1/4 cup tomato, chopped and seeded

1 tablespoon low-fat Cheddar cheese, shredded

salt and ground black pepper, to taste

> Coat a skillet or frying pan in cooking spray and place over medium-high heat. Add the mushrooms, peppers, and onions; continue to sauté until onions are translucent.

> In a large mixing bowl, whisk together the eggs and skim milk. Add the egg mixture to the vegetables and stir. Add the tomatoes and continue to stir. Cook until the eggs are almost done, then sprinkle on the cheese, salt, and pepper.

TASTY TURKEY & SPINACH OMELET

1/2 cup onions, chopped

1/2 cup mushrooms, sliced

3 ounces deli turkey slices, chopped

6 egg whites

1 large egg

1 slice fat-free cheese

1 cup spinach

Servings	1
Prep Time	5 mins
Cooking Time	10 mins

PER SERVING

Calories	315
Protein	49 grams
Carbohydrates	13 grams
Fat	8 grams

> Lightly coat a nonstick pan with cooking spray and place over medium heat. Add the onion, mushrooms, and turkey and cook for about 5 minutes. Once cooked, transfer to a plate and set aside.

> Mix the egg and egg whites in a bowl and pour the mixture into the pan.

> After a couple of minutes, you should see bubbles. Gently lift the edges of the omelet with a spatula to let the uncooked part of the eggs flow toward the edges and cook. Continue cooking for 2 – 3 minutes or until the center of the omelet starts to look dry.

> Place the slice of fat-free cheese in the middle of the omelet and spread the turkey mixture and spinach on top (in the center of the omelet). Using a spatula gently fold one edge of the omelet over.

> Let the omelet cook for another two minutes or until the cheese melts to your desired consistency. Slide the omelet out of the skillet and onto a plate.

BREAKFAST BAKING

When you think of getting ripped, you don't think of muffins, biscuits, and bread. And rightly so—pre-made foods like these are full of unhealthy carbs, sugar, and fats, and they're usually full of sodium too. But boy, do they taste good. What are we to do?

Simple. Make your own, and make them healthy. These recipes are tweaked to do your body good with whole-grain flour, protein powder, flaxseed oil, and egg whites.

BANANA MASH MUSCLE MUFFINS

Servings	3 (1 muffin per serving)
Prep Time	10 mins
Cooking Time	15 – 20 mins

PER SERVING

Calories	271
Protein	17 grams
Carbohydrates	32 grams
Fat	11 grams

3/4 cup old-fashioned oats

1/4 cup oat bran

1 tablespoon whole grain flour

1/2 teaspoon ground cinnamon

1/2 scoop chocolate whey protein powder

1/4 teaspoon baking soda

6 egg whites

1/2 teaspoon stevia or other sugar alternative

1 tablespoon flaxseed oil

1 large ripe banana, mashed

2 tablespoons walnuts, chopped

> Preheat the oven to 400°F.

> In a large bowl, combine the first six ingredients. In a separate bowl, beat the eggs, stevia, and oil. Stir the dry ingredients in until just moistened. Fold in the mashed bananas and nuts, careful not to mix too much.

> Lightly coat a nonstick muffin pan with cooking spray and pour in the mixture (each cup should only be 3/4 full). Bake for about 15 – 18 minutes, until the tops are golden and a toothpick inserted into the middle comes out clean. Let them sit for a few minutes before removing them from the pan.

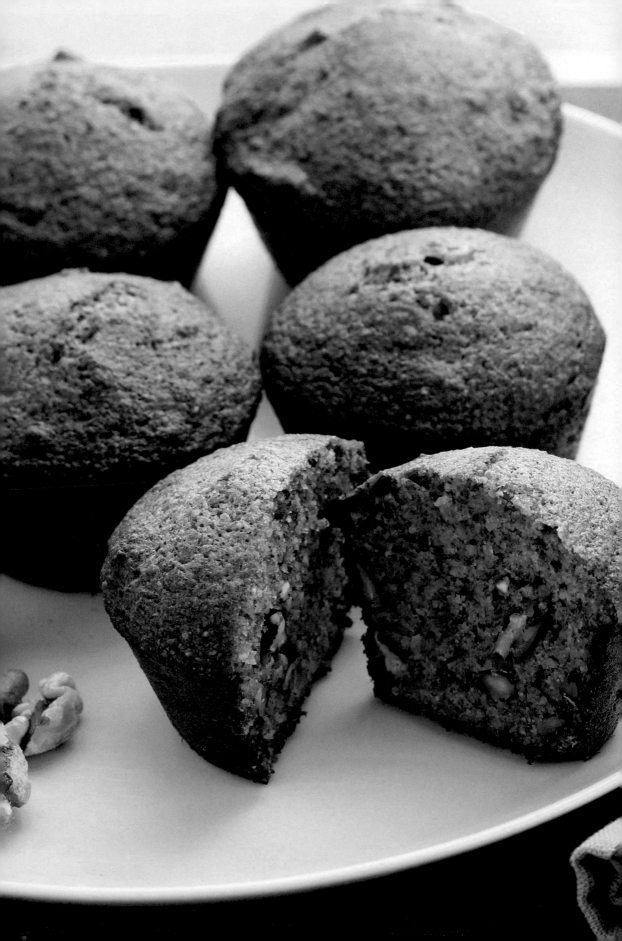

MAPLE WALNUT PROTEIN MUFFINS

Servings	12
Prep Time	10 mins
Cooking Time	15 – 20 mins

PER SERVING

Calories	179
Protein	16 grams
Carbohydrates	13 grams
Fat	8 grams

3 egg whites

3 tablespoons walnut oil or unsalted butter, softened

1/4 cup maple syrup

1/2 cup skim milk

1/2 cup whole grain flour

1/4 cup wheat germ

1/4 cup oat bran

6 scoops chocolate whey protein powder

2 teaspoons baking powder

1 teaspoon baking soda

1/2 cup chopped walnuts

> Preheat the oven to 350°F.

> In a large mixing bowl, add the egg whites, oil, maple syrup, and skim milk and mix well. In a separate bowl, mix together the flour, wheat germ, oat bran, protein powder, baking powder, and baking soda. Combine the dry and wet ingredients, stir only until the dry ingredients are moistened. Gently stir in the nuts.

> Lightly coat a nonstick muffin pan with cooking spray and pour in the mixture (each cup should only be 3/4 full). Bake for 20 – 25 minutes or until toasty brown and a toothpick inserted into the middle comes out clean. Let them sit for a few minutes before removing them from the pan.

MIXED BERRY MUFFINS

Servings	10 (1 muffin per serving)
Prep Time	5 mins
Cooking Time	15 – 20 mins

PER SERVING

Calories	165
Protein	18 grams
Carbohydrates	19 grams
Fat	2 grams

1 cup old-fashioned oats, finely blended

1 cup fat-free cottage cheese

1 tablespoon vanilla extract

8 egg whites

14 pitted dates

1/2 lemon, juiced

1/4 cup ground flaxseed

1/2 teaspoon cinnamon

4 scoops chocolate or vanilla whey protein powder

3/4 cup fresh or frozen mixed berries

> Preheat the oven to 400°F.

> Blend all the ingredients except the berries until it's a smooth batter. Gently fold the berries into the batter.

> Lightly coat a nonstick muffin pan with cooking spray and pour the batter evenly in the 10 cups (each cup should only be 3/4 full). Bake for about 16 minutes or until cooked. The tops should be golden and a toothpick inserted into the middle should come out clean. Let them sit for a few minutes before removing them from the pan.

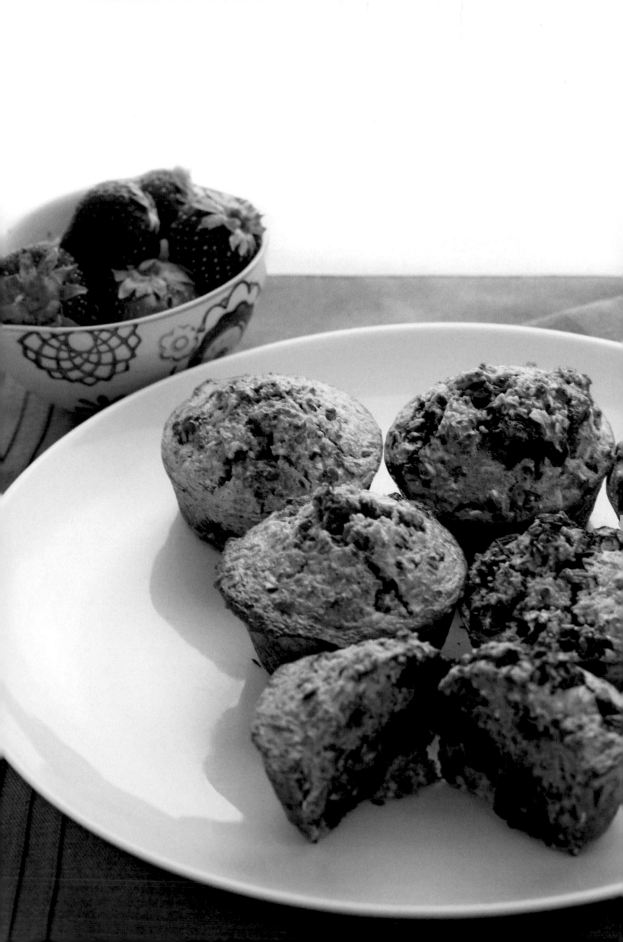

SWEET POTATO MUFFINS

Servings	8 (1 muffin per serving)
Prep Time	5 mins
Cooking Time	20 mins

PER SERVING

Calories	110
Protein	15 grams
Carbohydrates	11 grams
Fat	1 gram

2 medium sized sweet potatoes, cooked and peeled

1/2 cup old-fashioned oats

4 scoops chocolate or vanilla protein powder

1 tablespoon stevia or other sugar alternative

2 egg whites

1/2 teaspoon cinnamon

1/2 teaspoon vanilla extract

1 teaspoon baking powder

> Preheat the oven to 350°F.

> In a blender or food processor, add all of the ingredients. Blend until smooth.

> Lightly coat a nonstick muffin pan with cooking spray and pour in the mixture (each cup should only be 3/4 full). Bake for about 20 minutes or until cooked. The tops should be golden and a toothpick inserted into the middle should come out clean. Let them sit for a few minutes before removing from the pan.

CHICKEN & TURKEY

Like anyone who is into working out, I've come to love chicken and turkey. They're relatively cheap, super lean, full of protein, and they can be made to taste many different ways (and turkey can replace ground beef in many different recipes like meat loaf, chili, spaghetti sauce, hamburgers, and meatballs).

Turkey and chicken also make great "fast food." You can cook up a whole batch and keep it in the fridge. When you're in a hurry, grab about 5 ounces and an apple, and there's a quick meal.

CHICKEN & TURKEY RECIPES FOR GETTING BIG

MEXICAN MEATLOAF

Servings	8
Prep Time	5 – 10 mins
Cooking Time	50 mins – 1 hr

PER SERVING

Calories	285
Protein	32 grams
Carbohydrates	36 grams
Fat	3 grams

1 pound lean ground turkey

1 pound lean ground chicken

1 can (15 ounces) black beans, rinsed and drained

1 can (15 ounces) whole kernel corn, drained and rinsed

1/2 can (4 ounces) fire-roasted diced green chilis

1 cup mild chunky salsa

1 package (1 ounce) dry taco seasoning mix

3/4 cup plain bread crumbs

3 egg whites

1 can (28 ounces) enchilada sauce, divided

salt and ground black pepper to taste

> Preheat the oven to 400°F. Coat a 9 x 13 inch baking dish with cooking spray.

> In a large mixing bowl, combine the ground turkey, ground chicken, black beans, corn, green chilies, salsa, taco seasoning, bread crumbs, and egg whites and mix thoroughly.

> Form the mixture into a loaf shape and place inside the prepared baking dish, top with half of the enchilada sauce and place in the oven for 45 minutes.

> Remove from the oven and top with the remaining enchilada sauce, return to the oven and bake until the meatloaf is no longer pink inside, about 10 – 15 minutes. A thermometer inserted into the center should read at least 160°F.

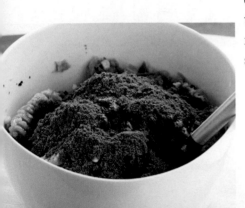

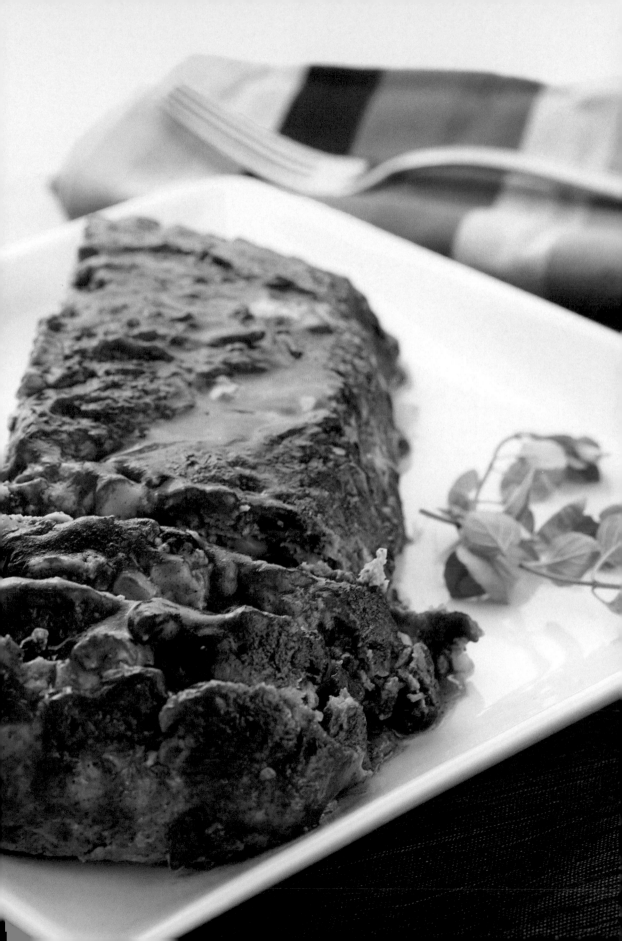

CHUNKY CHICKEN QUESADILLAS

Servings	2
Prep Time	Under 5 mins
Cooking Time	15 mins

PER SERVING

Calories	293
Protein	28 grams
Carbohydrates	31 grams
Fat	6 grams

1 boneless, skinless chicken breast (6 ounces), rinsed, dried, trimmed of fat

1 tablespoon fat-free sour cream

2 (8 inch) whole wheat tortillas

1/3 cup salsa

1 cup lettuce, shredded

1/3 cup low-fat cheddar cheese, shredded

> Coat a medium-sized skillet with cooking spray and place over medium heat. Place chicken on the skillet and cook for 3 – 5 minutes per side, or until cooked through. Remove from heat and set aside.

> Spread the sour cream on one tortilla. Slice the chicken breast and spread on top. Cover with salsa and lettuce.

> Sprinkle the cheddar cheese on top and cover with the other tortilla.

> Coat a large pan with cooking spray and cook the quesadilla on low heat for about 3 minutes on each side. Turn carefully with a large spatula.

POLLO FAJITAS

Servings	4 (1 fajita per serving)
Prep Time	5 mins
Cooking Time	10 mins

PER SERVING

Calories	371
Protein	45 grams
Carbohydrates	31 grams
Fat	8 grams

4 boneless, skinless chicken breasts (6 ounces each), rinsed, dried, trimmed of fat, and cut into strips

1 tablespoon Worcestershire sauce

1 tablespoon apple cider vinegar

1 tablespoon low-sodium soy sauce

1 teaspoon chili powder

1 clove garlic, minced

1 dash hot sauce

1 tablespoon vegetable oil

1 medium onion, thinly sliced

1 green bell pepper, sliced

salt and ground black pepper, to taste

4 (8 inch) whole wheat tortillas

1/2 lemon, juiced

> In a medium-sized mixing bowl, add the Worcestershire sauce, vinegar, soy sauce, chili powder, garlic, and hot sauce. Add the chicken strips to the sauce and lightly mix to coat. Cover and let marinate at room temperature for 30 minutes (can also be refrigerated for several hours)

> Place the oil in a large skillet over high heat. Once the oil is hot, add the chicken strip mixture to the pan and sauté for 5 – 6 minutes. Add the onion and green pepper, season with salt and pepper, and continue to sauté for another 3 – 4 minutes, or until chicken is fully cooked.

> Warm the tortillas on a pan or in the microwave. Top tortillas with the fajita mixture, sprinkle with lemon juice.

AUSSIE CHICKEN

Servings	4
Prep Time	30 mins
Cooking Time	25 – 30 mins

PER SERVING

Calories	437
Protein	48 grams
Carbohydrates	20 grams
Fat	19 grams

4 boneless, skinless chicken breasts (6 ounces each), rinsed, dried, trimmed of fat and pounded to 1/2-inch thickness

2 teaspoons seasoning salt

6 slices bacon, cut in half

1/4 cup yellow mustard

1/4 cup honey

1/8 cup mayonnaise

1 tablespoon dried onion flakes

1 tablespoon vegetable oil

1 cup fresh mushrooms, sliced

1/2 cup reduced fat Monterey Jack cheese, shredded

2 tablespoons fresh parsley, chopped

> After prepping your chicken breasts, rub with the seasoning salt, cover and refrigerate for 30 minutes.

> Preheat the oven to 350°F.

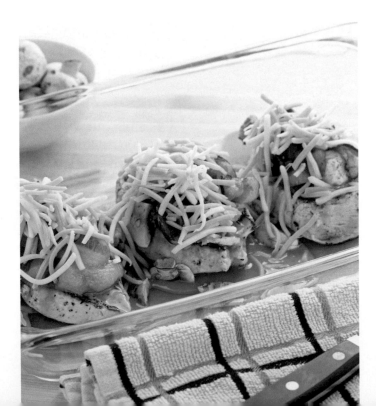

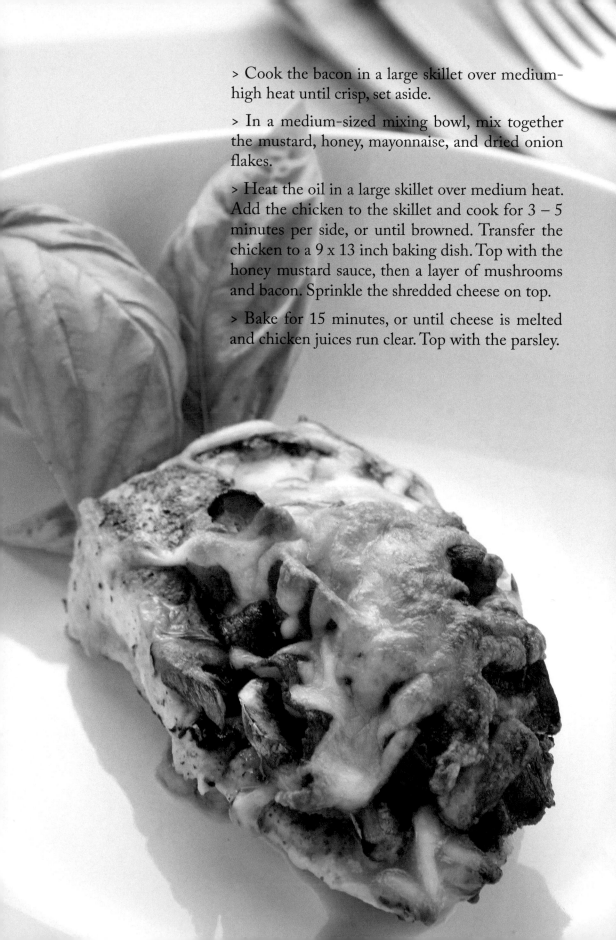

> Cook the bacon in a large skillet over medium-high heat until crisp, set aside.

> In a medium-sized mixing bowl, mix together the mustard, honey, mayonnaise, and dried onion flakes.

> Heat the oil in a large skillet over medium heat. Add the chicken to the skillet and cook for 3 – 5 minutes per side, or until browned. Transfer the chicken to a 9 x 13 inch baking dish. Top with the honey mustard sauce, then a layer of mushrooms and bacon. Sprinkle the shredded cheese on top.

> Bake for 15 minutes, or until cheese is melted and chicken juices run clear. Top with the parsley.

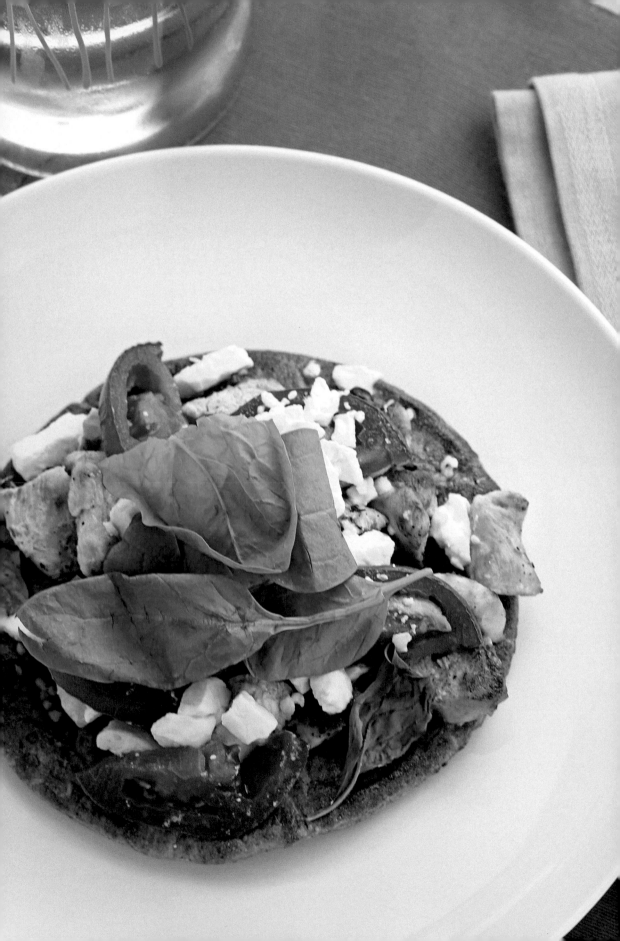

GREEK PITA PIZZA

Servings	1
Prep Time	5 mins
Cooking Time	10 – 15 mins

PER SERVING

Calories	472
Protein	49 grams
Carbohydrates	36 grams
Fat	15 grams

1 boneless, skinless chicken breast (6 ounces), rinsed, dried, trimmed of fat

1 whole grain pita bread

1/2 tablespoon extra-virgin olive oil

2 tablespoons olives, sliced

1 teaspoon red wine vinegar

1/2 clove garlic, minced

1/4 teaspoon dried oregano

1/4 teaspoon dried basil

salt and ground black pepper, to taste

1/4 cup fresh spinach

2 tablespoons low-fat feta cheese, crumbled

1/2 small tomato, chopped and seeded

> Coat a medium-sized skillet with cooking spray and place over medium heat. Place chicken on the skillet and cook for 3 – 5 minutes per side or until cooked through. Remove from heat and set aside.

> Prepare your pizza by brushing the pita with the oil. Place on a baking sheet and broil 4 inches from the heat for 2 minutes. Meanwhile, get a mixing bowl and add the olives, vinegar, garlic, oregano, basil, salt, pepper, and any remaining oil. Mix well.

> Spread the mixture over the pita. Chop the chicken breast into slices. Top the pita with the spinach, feta, tomato, and chopped chicken. Broil for about 3 more minutes, or until the cheese is desired consistency.

HARVEST CHICKEN STEW

Servings	6
Prep Time	15 mins
Cooking Time	1 hr – 1 hr 10 mins

PER SERVING

Calories	342
Protein	45 grams
Carbohydrates	35 grams
Fat	3 grams

6 boneless, skinless chicken breasts (6 ounces each), rinsed, dried, trimmed of fat, and cut into cubes

4 cups peeled eggplant, cut into 1-inch cubes

4 cups small red potatoes, cut into 1/8-inch slices

4 medium carrots, sliced

3 medium onions, cut into quarters

3 1/2 cups low-sodium chicken broth

3/4 cup fresh parsley, chopped

2 tablespoons fresh thyme leaves, chopped

1/4 teaspoon salt

1/4 teaspoon ground black pepper

1/2 cup cold water

2 tablespoons whole grain flour

> Preheat the oven to 350°F.

> Add the chicken, eggplant, potatoes, carrots, onions, broth, parsley, thyme, salt, and pepper to an ovenproof Dutch oven, cover and bake 50 minutes.

> Place the cold water and flour in a tightly covered container or sealable bag and shake. Add the flour mixture and the remaining ingredients to the stew and stir well. Cover and place back in oven for about 20 minutes longer, or until the potatoes are tender and chicken is fully cooked.

CHICKEN & TURKEY RECIPES FOR GETTING LEAN

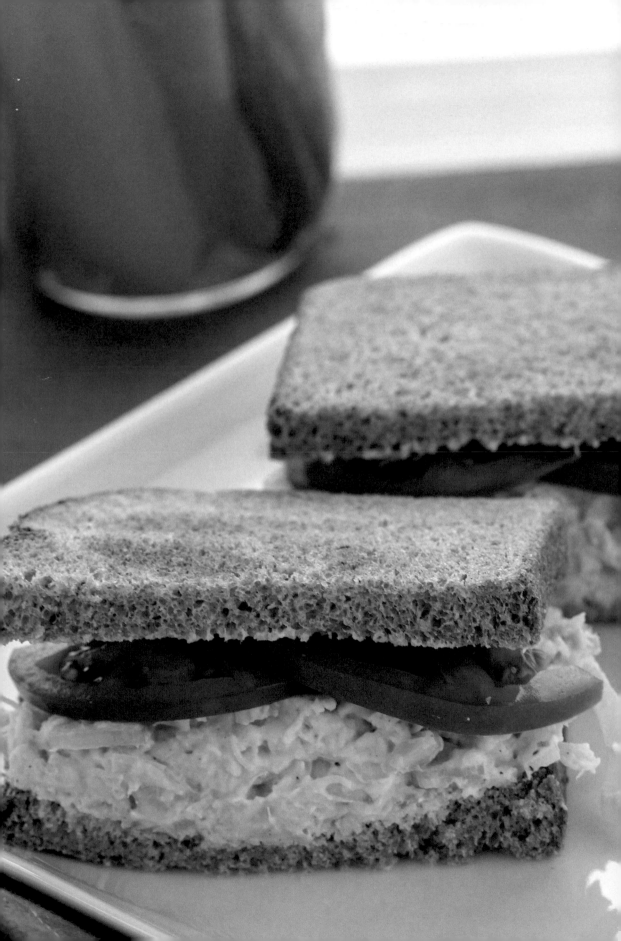

SUPER-FAST CHICKEN SALAD SANDWICH

Servings	2
Prep Time	5 mins
PER SERVING	
Calories	299
Protein	30 grams
Carbohydrates	30 grams
Fat	7 grams

2 cans (3 ounces each) chunk chicken, rinsed and drained twice

1 celery stick, finely chopped

1 tablespoon onion, finely chopped

1 tablespoon pine nuts

1 heaping teaspoon spicy brown mustard

1 heaping teaspoon fat-free sour cream

1 heaping teaspoon fat-free plain yogurt

pinch of ground black pepper

4 slices whole grain bread

2 leaves lettuce

> In a bowl, mix the celery, onion, pine nuts, mustard, sour cream, yogurt, and pepper. Mix in the chicken.

> Spread half of the mixture on a slice of bread. Top with a lettuce leaf and then with another slice of bread. Repeat with the rest of the mixture to make a second sandwich.

PINEAPPLE CHICKEN

Servings	2
Prep Time	3 – 5 mins
Cooking Time	10 mins

PER SERVING

Calories	342
Protein	40 grams
Carbohydrates	35 grams
Fat	5 grams

2 boneless, skinless chicken breasts (6 ounces each), rinsed, dried, trimmed of fat, and cut into small cubes

1 teaspoon extra-virgin olive oil

1/4 cup sweet onion, finely chopped

pinch of ground black pepper

1 tablespoon orange juice

1 can (8 ounces) pineapple chunks

1 banana, sliced

1 teaspoon maple syrup

> Put the oil in a pan and cook the onion on medium-high heat. Add the dash of pepper and cook for 1 minute, until the onion is slightly translucent.

> Put the chicken, orange juice, and pineapple with juice into the pan. Bring to a boil and reduce to medium heat.

> Add the banana and syrup and cook for 1 – 2 minutes.

> Stir it up and reduce the heat to low. Cover it and let it simmer for about 5 – 7 minutes, or until chicken is cooked through.

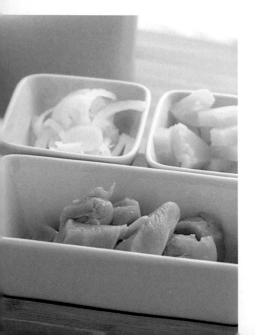

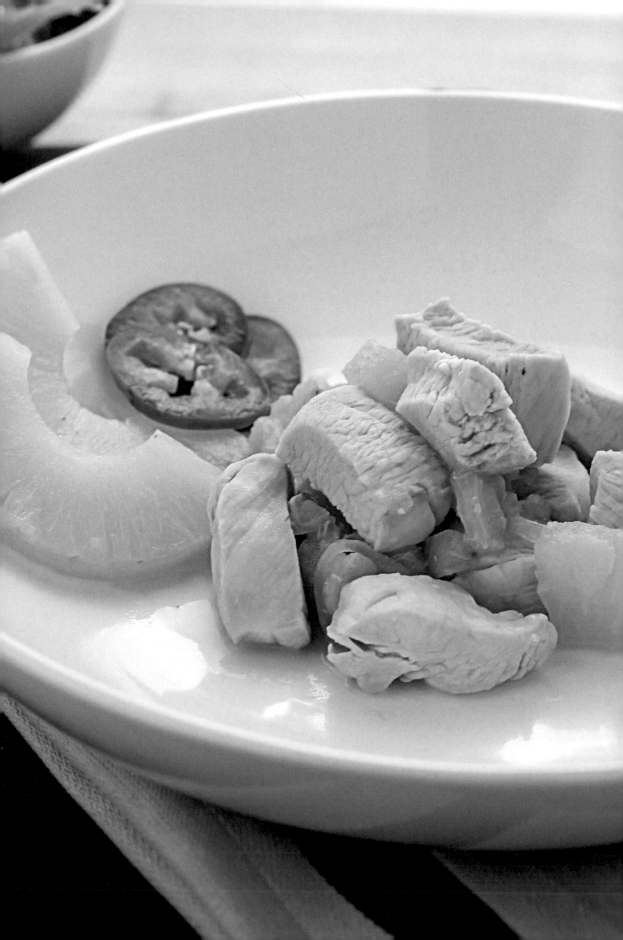

CHICKEN YAKITORI

Servings	4
Prep Time	5 mins
Cooking Time	10 – 15 mins

PER SERVING

Calories	253
Protein	41 grams
Carbohydrates	8 grams
Fat	2 grams

4 boneless, skinless chicken breasts (6 ounces each), rinsed, dried, trimmed of fat, cut into 2-inch cubes

1/2 cup low-sodium soy sauce

1/2 cup sherry or white cooking wine

1/2 cup low-sodium chicken broth

1/3 teaspoon ground ginger

1 pinch garlic powder

1/2 cup scallions, chopped

> Place a small saucepan over medium-high heat. Add the soy sauce, sherry, chicken broth, ginger, garlic powder, and scallions. Bring to a boil and immediately remove from heat, set aside.

> Preheat the oven's broiler. Start threading the chicken onto metal or bamboo skewers (if using wood, I recommend soaking in water for 30 minutes to prevent them catching on fire). Coat a broiler pan with cooking spray and place chicken skewers on pan. Brush each skewer with the sherry sauce.

> Place the pan under the broiler for 3 minutes, until browned. Remove from the oven, turn the chicken over and spoon a little more sauce onto each one. Return to the broiler until the chicken is cooked through and nicely browned.

HONEY GLAZED CHICKEN

Servings	4
Prep Time	5 – 10 mins
Cooking Time	25 – 30 mins
PER SERVING	
Calories	199
Protein	40 grams
Carbohydrates	10 grams
Fat	1 gram

4 boneless, skinless chicken breasts (6 ounces each), rinsed, dried, trimmed of fat

2 tablespoons orange juice

2 tablespoons honey

1 tablespoon lemon juice

1/8 teaspoon salt

> Preheat oven to 375°F.

> Coat a 9 x 13 inch baking dish with cooking spray, add the chicken. In a small mixing bowl, mix together the orange juice, honey, lemon juice, and salt. Baste each piece of chicken.

> Cover the dish with foil and bake for 10 minutes. Remove the foil and flip the chicken. Bake another 10 – 15 minutes, until the chicken is cooked through and the juices run clear.

MUSCLE MEATBALLS

Servings	4 (4 meatballs per serving)
Prep Time	10 mins
Cooking Time	20 – 25 mins

PER SERVING

Calories	266
Protein	46 grams
Carbohydrates	11 grams
Fat	5 grams

1 1/2 pounds extra-lean ground turkey breast

2 egg whites

1/2 cup toasted wheat germ

1/4 cup quick cooking oats

1 tablespoon whole flaxseeds

1 tablespoon Parmesan cheese, grated

1/2 teaspoon all-purpose seasoning

1/4 teaspoon ground black pepper

> Preheat the oven to 400°F. Coat a large baking dish with cooking spray.

> Mix all of the ingredients in a bowl.

> Make 16 meatballs and place them in the baking dish.

> Bake for 7 minutes and turn the meatballs. Bake for 8 – 13 minutes longer, or until no longer pink in the center.

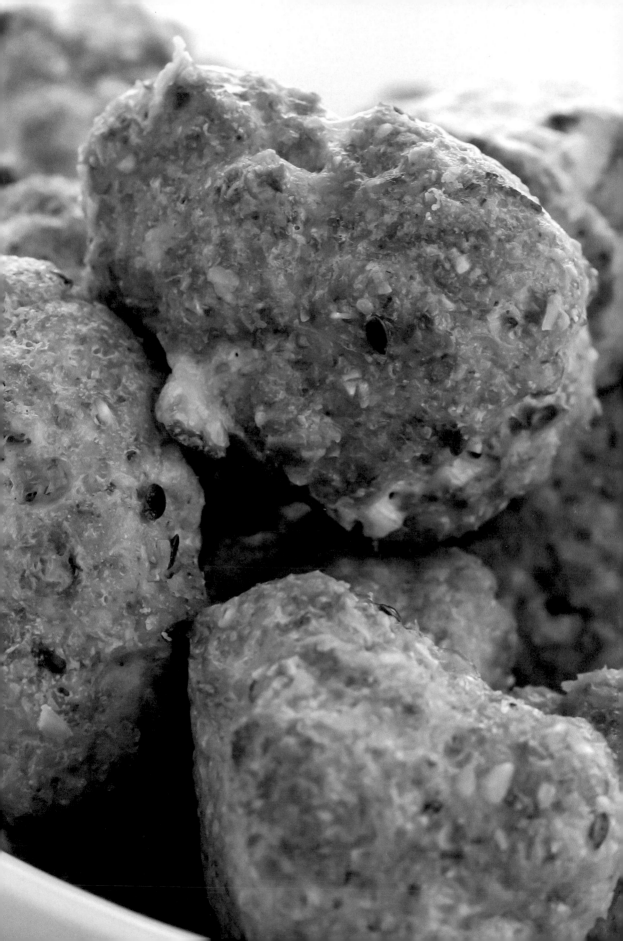

ANTIPASTO CHICKEN

Servings	4
Prep Time	5 mins
Cooking Time	20 – 25 mins
PER SERVING	
Calories	248
Protein	43 grams
Carbohydrates	8 grams
Fat	6 grams

4 boneless, skinless chicken breasts (6 ounces each), rinsed, dried, trimmed of fat

1 teaspoon garlic-pepper blend

1 jar (6 ounces) marinated artichoke hearts, undrained

1 small red bell pepper, chopped

2 medium tomatoes, chopped

1 can (2 1/4 ounces) ripe olives, drained and sliced

1 tablespoon fresh basil, chopped

> Coat a 12-inch skillet in cooking spray and place over medium heat. Sprinkle the chicken breasts with the garlic-pepper blend and place in skillet.

> Cook for about 3 – 5 minutes, flip, and cook another 3 – 5 minutes, until brown.

> In a medium-sized mixing bowl, mix together the remaining ingredients (depending on the artichoke hearts you get, they may need to be cut in half). Spoon the mixture over the chicken and continue to sauté, about 10 minutes longer, or until the chicken is cooked through.

THAI BASIL CHICKEN

4 boneless, skinless chicken breasts (6 ounces each), rinsed, dried, trimmed of fat

3 cloves garlic, finely chopped

2 jalapeño peppers, seeded and finely chopped

1 tablespoon fish sauce

1 teaspoon stevia or other sugar alternative

1/4 cup fresh basil, chopped

1 tablespoon fresh mint, chopped

1 tablespoon unsalted dry-roasted peanuts, chopped

Servings	4
Prep Time	5 mins
Cooking Time	10 – 15 mins

PER SERVING

Calories	191
Protein	41 grams
Carbohydrates	2 grams
Fat	3 grams

> Cut each chicken breast into about 8 strips, set aside.

> Coat a 12-inch skillet in cooking spray and heat over medium-high heat. Add the garlic and chiles and sauté, stirring constantly until garlic is just golden.

> Add the chicken strips and cook 8 – 10 minutes, stirring frequently, until chicken is cooked through. Add the fish sauce and stevia and sauté 30 seconds. Remove from heat and sprinkle on the basil, mint, and peanuts.

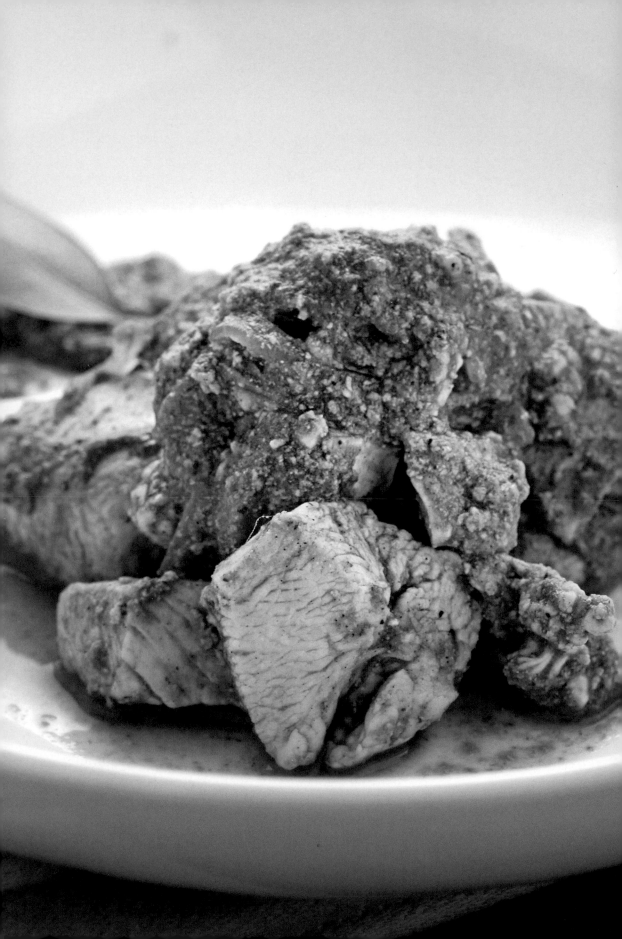

INDIAN CURRY CHICKEN

Servings	4
Prep Time	10 mins
Cooking Time	20 – 25 mins

PER SERVING

Calories	247
Protein	46 grams
Carbohydrates	9 grams
Fat	3 grams

4 boneless, skinless chicken breasts (6 ounces each), rinsed, dried, trimmed of fat, cut into 1-inch cubes

1 small onion, chopped

1 clove garlic, minced

3 tablespoons curry powder

1 teaspoon paprika

1 bay leaf

1 teaspoon ground cinnamon

1/2 teaspoon fresh ginger root, grated

salt and ground black pepper, to taste

1 tablespoon tomato paste

1 cup fat-free plain Greek yogurt

1/2 cup water

1/2 lemon, juiced

1/2 teaspoon Indian chili powder

> Coat a 12-inch skillet with cooking spray and place over medium heat. Sauté the onion until translucent, then stir in the garlic, curry powder, paprika, bay leaf, cinnamon, ginger, salt, and pepper.

> Continue stirring for 2 minutes, then add in the chicken, tomato paste, yogurt, and water. Bring to a boil, then reduce heat and simmer for 10 minutes. Remove the bay leaf, stir in the lemon juice and chili powder. Simmer 5 more minutes, or until chicken is cooked through.

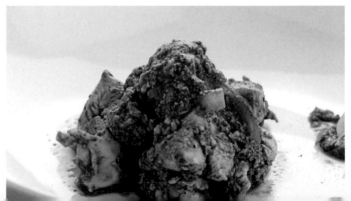

SIMPLE ITALIAN CHICKEN

Servings	4
Prep Time	5 mins
Cooking Time	20 – 25 mins
PER SERVING	
Calories	281
Protein	40 grams
Carbohydrates	5 grams
Fat	12 grams

4 boneless, skinless chicken breasts (6 ounces each), rinsed, dried, trimmed of fat

2 tablespoons extra-virgin olive oil   4.5

2 teaspoons garlic, crushed   4.5

1/4 cup seasoned bread crumbs   .6

1/4 cup low-fat Parmesan cheese, grated   .6

> Preheat the oven to 425°F.

> Warm the olive oil and garlic in the microwave to blend the flavors. In a separate bowl, combine the bread crumbs and Parmesan cheese. Dredge the chicken breasts in the oil mixture, letting the excess run off, then coat in the bread crumb mixture.

> Place the coated chicken breasts into a shallow baking dish and place in the oven for 10 minutes, flip and cook for another 10 – 15 minutes, until the chicken is no longer pink in the center and the juices run clear.

GRILLED GINGER CHICKEN

Servings	4
Prep Time	5 mins
Cooking Time	10 – 15 mins
PER SERVING	
Calories	247
Protein	41 grams
Carbohydrates	5 grams
Fat	9 grams

4 boneless, skinless chicken breasts (6 ounces each), rinsed, dried, trimmed of fat

2 tablespoons canola oil

1/4 cup low-sodium soy sauce

3 lemons, juiced

1/4 teaspoon garlic powder

1 teaspoon onion salt

1 tablespoon ground ginger

> In a small mixing bowl, combine the oil, soy sauce, lemon juice, garlic powder, onion salt, and ground ginger. Place the chicken in a ziplock bag and pour the marinade in. Seal tightly and place in refrigerator to marinate for at least 4 hours.

> Grill over direct medium heat for about 4 – 5 minutes, turn and cook for another 4 – 5 minutes, or until chicken is cooked through.

CHICKEN & VEGETABLE STIR-FRY

4 boneless, skinless chicken breasts (6 ounces each), rinsed, dried, trimmed of fat, cut into thin strips

2 tablespoons red wine

1 tablespoon low-sodium soy sauce

1/2 teaspoon cornstarch

1 teaspoon stevia or other sugar alternative

1 teaspoon salt

2 cups broccoli florets

1 red bell pepper, seeded and chopped

1/2 cup yellow onion, sliced

Servings	4
Prep Time	5 mins
Cooking Time	15 mins

PER SERVING

Calories	200
Protein	42 grams
Carbohydrates	6 grams
Fat	2 grams

> In a small mixing bowl, combine the red wine, soy sauce, cornstarch, stevia, and salt. Mix well to dissolve the cornstarch.

> Coat a 12-inch skillet in cooking spray and place over medium-high heat. Add the broccoli, bell pepper, and onion. Sauté until the vegetables are tender and onions are browned. Add the chicken and stir-fry for 2 – 3 more minutes, until chicken is browned.

> Pour the sauce over the chicken and vegetables and continue to stir-fry until sauce is thickened and chicken is cooked through, about 2 – 4 minutes.

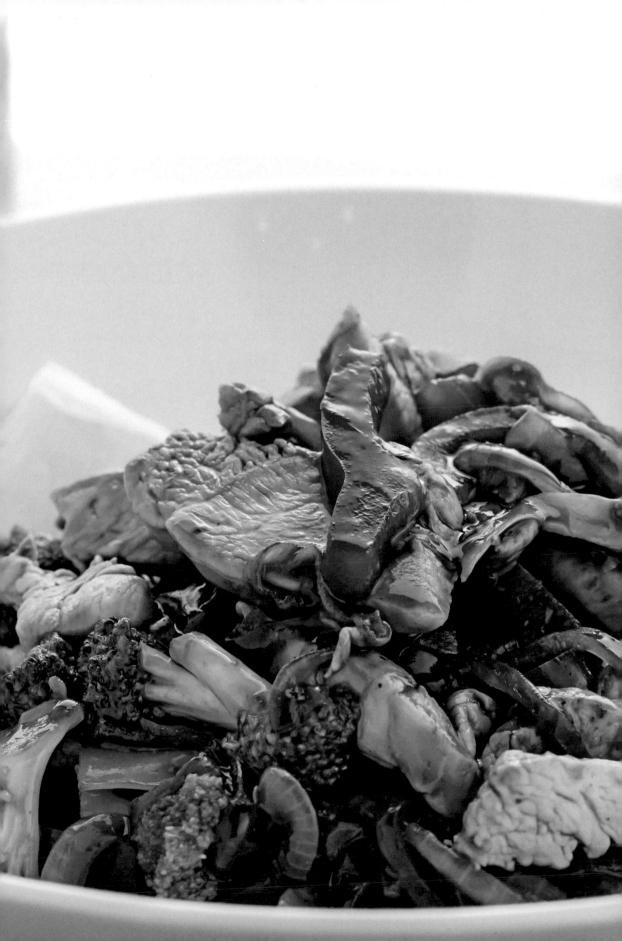

CHICKEN STROGANOFF

Servings	4
Prep Time	5 mins
Cooking Time	15 – 20 mins
PER SERVING	
Calories	245
Protein	50 grams
Carbohydrates	11 grams
Fat	3 grams

4 boneless, skinless chicken breasts (6 ounces each), rinsed, dried, trimmed of fat, sliced

salt and ground black pepper, to taste

1 medium onion, chopped

2 tablespoons garlic, minced

2 tablespoons dried tarragon

2 1/2 cups fresh mushrooms, sliced

3/4 cup low-sodium chicken broth

1/2 container (8 ounces) fat-free sour cream

> Coat a 12-inch skillet with cooking spray and place over medium-high heat. Add salt and pepper to your chicken breast and place into skillet. Cook until golden on one side, about 2 minutes, turn and repeat.

> Push the chicken pieces to one side of the skillet. Add the onion to the other side and sauté until softened. Stir in the garlic, tarragon, and mushrooms and cook for 2 more minutes.

> Add the chicken broth and stir, lower the heat to medium-low. Add the sour cream and mix the chicken in well with the rest of the sauce. Simmer for 5 minutes, stirring occasionally, until sauce slightly thickens.

5 DELICIOUS CHICKEN MARINADES

Below are five quick and easy marinades for chicken for changing up the tastes of any of the chicken recipes. To prepare each, simply put the ingredients in a bowl and mix.

The best way to marinate chicken is to put the marinade and chicken into a large ziplop sandwich bag and let it sit overnight in the fridge. These amounts are for 1 – 2 cups of marinade, good for 3 – 5 chicken breasts.

TERIYAKI

You can do this one in two ways. If you want to make it really easy, you can make a nice zesty teriyaki marinade by using 1/2 cup Italian dressing and 1/2 cup teriyaki sauce.

If you want to make teriyaki marinade from scratch it's as follows:

1/2 cup soy sauce

1/2 cup water

1/8 cup Worcestershire sauce

1 1/2 tablespoons distilled white vinegar

1 1/2 tablespoons vegetable oil

1 1/2 tablespoons onion powder

1 teaspoon garlic powder

1/2 teaspoon ginger powder

stevia to taste

PINEAPPLE

1 cup crushed pineapple

1/3 cup soy sauce

1/3 cup honey

1/4 cup cider vinegar

2 cloves garlic, minced

1 teaspoon ginger powder

1/4 teaspoon powdered cloves

LEMON-WINE

2 tablespoons olive oil

1/4 cup white wine

2 tablespoons fresh lemon juice

2 tablespoons brown sugar

1 tablespoon fresh thyme

1 tablespoon fresh rosemary

2 cloves garlic, minced

2 teaspoons lemon zest

CARNE ASADA

1/4 cups red wine vinegar

2 tablespoons olive oil

2 tablespoons steak sauce

1 clove garlic, minced

1 teaspoon sage

1 teaspoon savory

1/2 teaspoon salt

1/2 teaspoon dry mustard

1/2 teaspoon paprika

JALAPEÑO LIME

1/2 cup orange juice concentrate

1/3 cup chopped onion

1/4 cup lime juice

2 tablespoons honey

1/2 seeded and diced jalapeño pepper

1 teaspoon ground cumin

1 teaspoon grated lime peel

1/4 teaspoon garlic salt

1 clove garlic, minced

BEEF

It's hard to beat beef when it comes to muscle-building proteins, with every ounce giving you six grams of protein. It's high in creatine (an amino acid that helps with muscle repair and also boosts strength) and high in iron (which promotes healthy blood), and it contains a spectrum of other nutrients, such as vitamin B12, zinc, and antioxidants.

How lean do you want your beef? 80% lean or fattier is too fatty (ground chuck, for instance, has more fat per ounce than protein, which makes sticking to a reasonable diet tough). Look for the "extra lean" or "select" category of meats, which have 15% fat or less. As long as you don't overcook these meats, they can taste great. I love making hamburgers from 95% lean beef with a nice red color. Some of the leanest cuts of beef are tenderloin, eye of round, top loin, sirloin tip, and bottom round.

I also highly recommend that you spend a little extra money to get hormone-free, cage-free, grass-fed beef. Run-of-the-mill meats come from cows that have been pumped full of antibiotics and steroids and fed with genetically modified crops covered in pesticides. Traces of all these chemicals make their way into your system when you eat the meat, and they can interfere with your body's natural balance of hormones.

Additionally, when an animal was raised in a cage, the food it produces is inferior to its free-roaming counterparts. Cage-free chickens produce healthier eggs higher in omega-3 fatty acids, and meat from free-roaming cows has significantly higher amounts of vitamin E and conjugated linoleic acid (a fat that promotes the growth of muscle and the reduction of fat) than meat from cattle cooped up in a pen.

The bottom line is that lean beef is an awesome testosterone-boosting, muscle-building source of protein, and you should absolutely include it in your diet.

BEEF RECIPES FOR GETTING BIG

KOREAN BBQ BEEF

Servings	4
Prep Time	5 mins
Cooking Time	Under 5 mins

PER SERVING

Calories	307
Protein	39 grams
Carbohydrates	6 grams
Fat	13 grams

1 1/2 pounds lean flank steak, thinly sliced

1/3 cup low-sodium soy sauce

1 tablespoon stevia or other sugar alternative

1/4 cup scallions, chopped

2 tablespoons garlic, minced

2 tablespoons sesame seeds

1 tablespoon sesame oil

1/2 teaspoon ground black pepper

> In a small mixing bowl, combine the soy sauce, stevia, scallions, garlic, sesame seeds, sesame oil, and ground black pepper. Mix well.

> Place the beef in a large ziplock bag or container, pour the soy sauce marinade over it and seal. Refrigerate for at least 1 hour.

> Lightly coat a large skillet in cooking spray and place over high heat. Add the beef and sauté until cooked through, 1 – 2 minutes per side.

MIKE'S SAVORY BURGERS

Servings	4
Prep Time	Under 5 mins
Cooking Time	10 – 15 mins

PER SERVING

Calories	395 grams
Protein	41 grams
Carbohydrates	32 grams
Fat	12 grams

1 1/2 pounds extra-lean ground round or chuck

4 tablespoons Dijon mustard

salt and ground black pepper, to taste

1/2 cup low-carb ketchup

1/2 cup low-fat mayonnaise

1 tablespoon red wine vinegar

2 teaspoons Worcestershire sauce

4 whole grain hamburger buns, toasted

4 sandwich slice pickles, halved

> Preheat a grill over high heat.

> In a large mixing bowl, combine the beef, mustard, salt, and pepper. Shape into 4 equal sized patties and grill, 5 – 6 minutes per side for medium doneness.

> Meanwhile, in a large mixing bowl, mix together the ketchup, mayo, vinegar, and Worcestershire sauce.

> Toast the buns by cutting in half and placing on the grill cut side down, for about 10 seconds. They should be light golden brown. Top each burger with pickles and sauce.

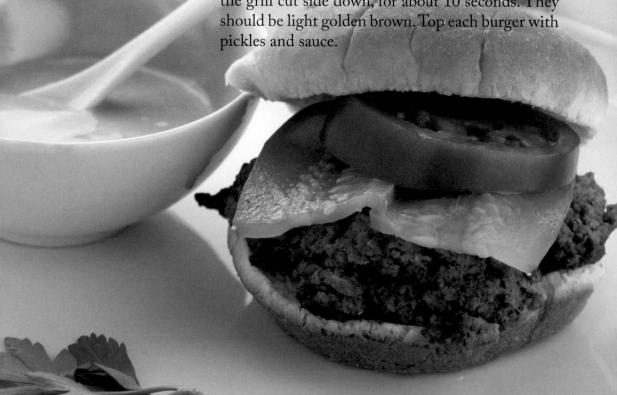

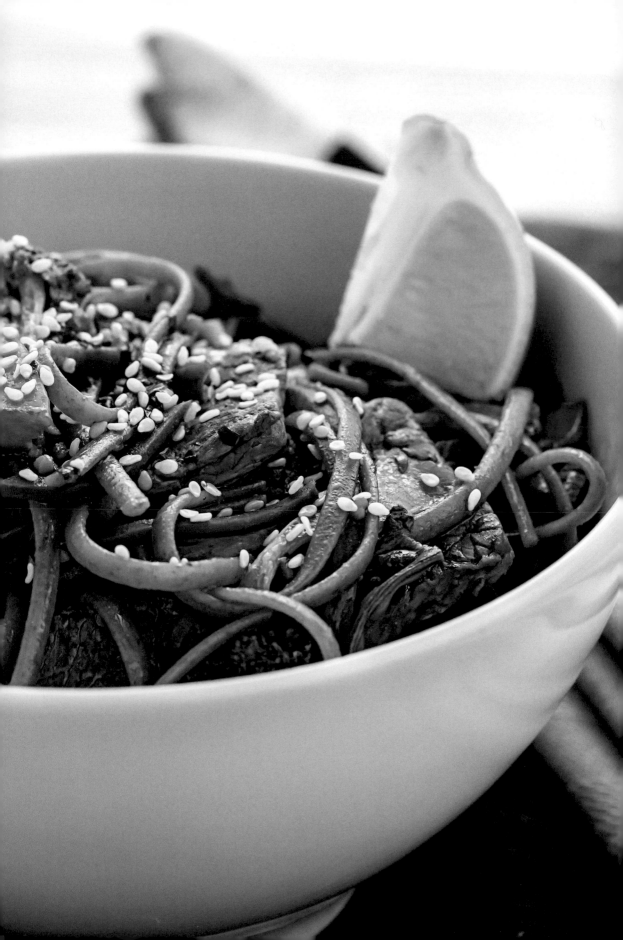

BEEF LO MEIN

6 ounces extra lean beef, sliced into 1-inch strips

1 teaspoon sesame oil

1/4 cup fresh snow pea pods, trimmed

1/4 cup broccoli florets

1/4 cup carrots, shredded

1 scallion, chopped

1/8 teaspoon red pepper flakes

1/2 garlic clove, minced

2 tablespoons low-sodium soy sauce

1/2 teaspoon fresh ginger, grated

2 ounces whole grain noodles, cooked

1 teaspoon sesame seeds, toasted

Servings	1
Prep Time	5 – 10 mins
Cooking Time	10 – 15 mins
PER SERVING	
Calories	526 grams
Protein	49 grams
Carbohydrates	45 grams
Fat	15 grams

> Heat the oil in a wok or large skillet over medium-high heat. Add the beef and stir-fry for 4 – 6 minutes or until browned. Remove from pan and set aside.

> Add the snow peas, broccoli, carrots, scallions, red pepper flakes, and garlic and stir-fry for 2 – 3 minutes. Add the soy sauce, ginger, cooked noodles, and beef. Mix together well and stir-fry until hot.

> Remove from heat and sprinkle with sesame seeds.

STEAK SOFT TACOS

Servings	4 (2 tacos per serving)
Prep Time	10 mins
Cooking Time	10 mins

PER SERVING

Calories	431
Protein	34 grams
Carbohydrates	56 grams
Fat	10 grams

12 ounces extra-lean strip steak, thinly sliced

1/2 teaspoon ground cumin

1 teaspoon chili powder

3 cloves garlic, minced

2 cups cooked black beans, drained

1 cup salsa

8 (6 inch) whole wheat tortillas

1 cup tomato, finely chopped

1/2 cup onion, finely chopped

1 cup shredded lettuce

8 teaspoons low-fat cheddar cheese, shredded

> Place the beef in a large mixing bowl, add the cumin, chili powder, and garlic and toss to coat.

> Coat a large skillet in cooking spray and place over medium-high heat. Add the steak and stir-fry for 4 – 6 minutes. Add the beans and salsa and stir-fry until desired doneness, then remove from heat.

> Meanwhile, warm the tortillas in a pan or the microwave. Top each tortilla with 1/8 of the steak mixture and toppings.

MOIST MEATLOAF

2 pounds extra-lean ground round or chuck

1 teaspoon salt

1/2 teaspoon ground black pepper

1 egg

1 cup stuffing mix

1/2 cup skim milk

1/3 cup steak sauce

1 onion, diced

1/2 medium green bell pepper, diced

Servings	6
Prep Time	5 – 10 mins
Cooking Time	50 mins – 1 hr
PER SERVING	
Calories	252
Protein	35 grams
Carbohydrates	11 grams
Fat	7 grams

> Preheat oven to 350°F. Lightly coat an 8.5 x 4.5 inch loaf pan.

> In a large mixing bowl, add the ground beef, salt, pepper, egg, and stuffing mix and thoroughly mix. Stir in the skim milk, 3 tablespoons of the steak sauce, onion, and bell pepper.

> Transfer the mixture to the baking pan and form into a loaf. Baste the top with the remaining steak sauce. Transfer to oven and bake for 1 hour.

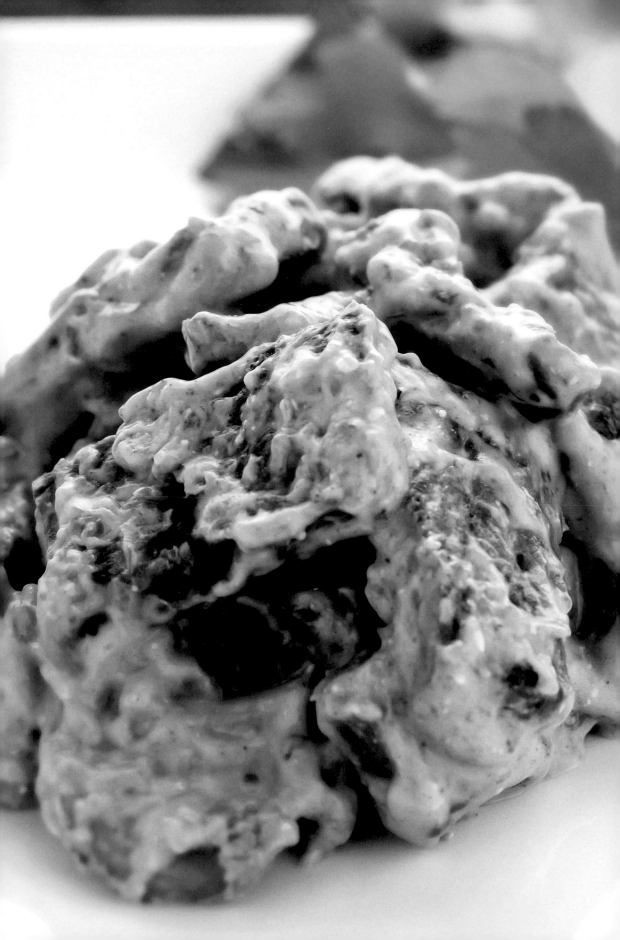

BEEF STROGANOFF

Servings	4
Prep Time	10 mins
Cooking Time	1 hr – 1 hr 10 mins
PER SERVING	
Calories	322
Protein	30 grams
Carbohydrates	9 grams
Fat	19 grams

1 pound lean beef tenderloin, sliced

1/4 teaspoon salt

1/4 teaspoon ground black pepper

4 tablespoons unsalted butter

1/2 medium yellow onion, sliced

2 tablespoons cornstarch

1/2 can (10.5 ounces) condensed beef broth

1/2 teaspoon Dijon mustard

1 clove garlic, minced

1/2 tablespoon Worcestershire sauce

1 can (4 ounces) sliced mushrooms, drained

3 tablespoons fat-free sour cream

3 tablespoons fat-free cream cheese

3 tablespoons white wine

> Season the meat with the salt and pepper. Melt the butter in a large skillet over medium heat. Add the beef and brown on all sides. Push to one side of the pan.

> Add the onions and cook for 3 – 5 minutes, until tender. Push the onions over to the side with the beef. Mix the cornstarch with 2 tablespoons of beef broth then pour into the skillet, mix with the juices in the pan to dissolve.

> Pour in the remaining beef broth. Bring to a boil, stirring frequently. Lower the heat and stir in the mustard, garlic, and Worcestershire. Cover with a tight fitting lid and simmer for 45 minutes to an hour, until the meat is a desired level of doneness.

> 5 minutes before the beef is done, stir in the mushrooms, sour cream, cream cheese, and white wine. Stir well and let the beef finish cooking in the sauce.

SUPREMELY SPICY CHILI

Servings	12
Prep Time	15 mins
Cooking Time	2 hrs

PER SERVING

Calories	474
Protein	44 grams
Carbohydrates	38 grams
Fat	15 grams

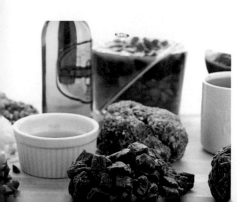

2 pounds extra-lean ground round

1 pound boneless chuck, trimmed of fat, and cut into 1/4-inch cubes

1 pound bulk Italian sausage

2 tablespoons unsalted butter

1 tablespoon canola oil

2 red bell peppers, diced

2 jalapeño peppers, finely chopped

3 Anaheim chilies, roasted, peeled, and chopped

3 poblano chilies, roasted, peeled, and chopped

2 yellow onions, diced

4 tablespoons garlic, minced

2 teaspoons granulated onion

2 teaspoons granulated garlic

3 tablespoons chili powder

2 teaspoons hot paprika

2 teaspoons ground cumin

2 teaspoons cayenne pepper

2 teaspoons ground coriander

2 teaspoons salt

2 teaspoons ground black pepper

1 cup tomato paste

2 cups tomato sauce

12 ounces lager beer

1 cup low-sodium chicken stock

2 cans (15.5 ounces) pinto beans, with juice

2 cans (15.5 ounces) kidney beans, with juice

1/2 cup scallions, thinly sliced

> Place a large stock pot or Dutch oven over high heat, add the butter and canola oil. Once butter has melted, add the bell pepper, jalapeño, chilies, and onion and cook until tender, about 5 minutes.

> Add the chuck cubes and brown on all sides. Mix in the ground round, sausage, and minced garlic, gently stir, trying not to break up the ground meat too much. Cook until meat is browned and cooked through, about 7 – 10 minutes.

> Stir in the granulated onions, granulated garlic, chili powder, paprika, cumin, cayenne, coriander, salt, and pepper and let cook for 1 minute. Stir in the tomato paste and sauce and let cook for 2 minutes. Pour in the beer, chicken stock, and beans. Thoroughly mix together, lower heat to medium-low and simmer for 2 hours, stirring occasionally. Serve with scallions on top.

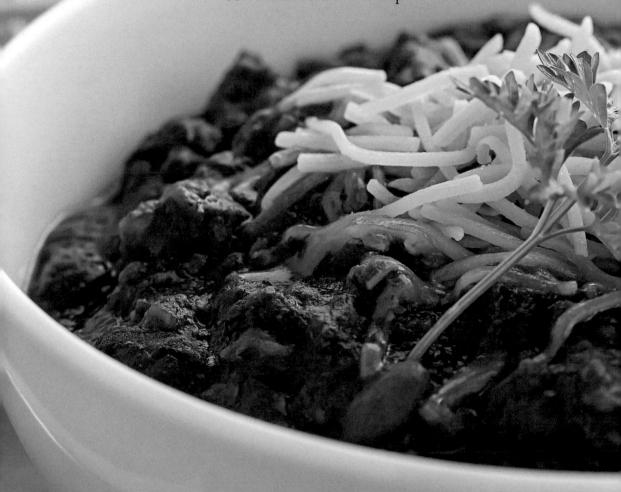

BEEF RECIPES FOR GETTING LEAN

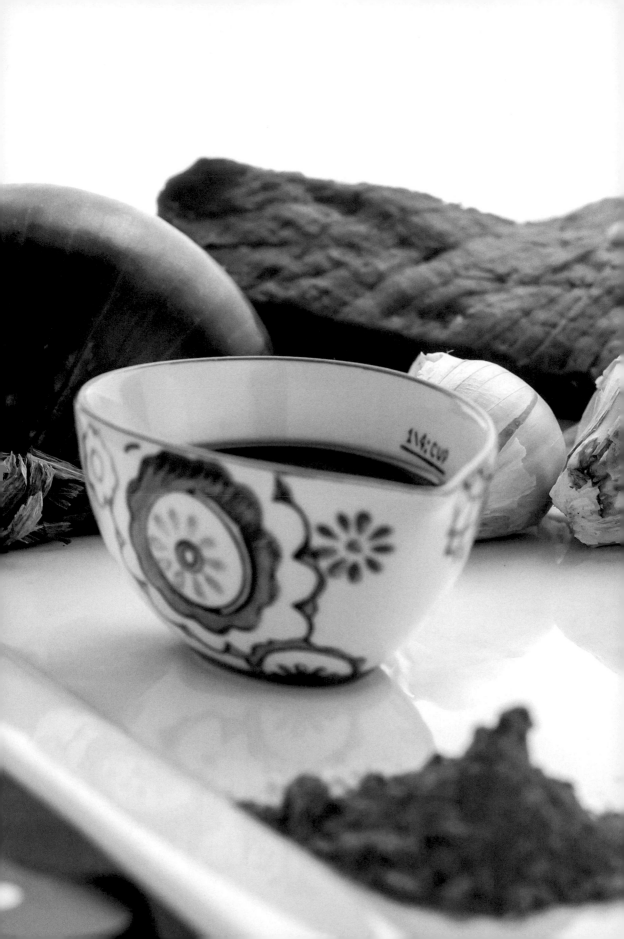

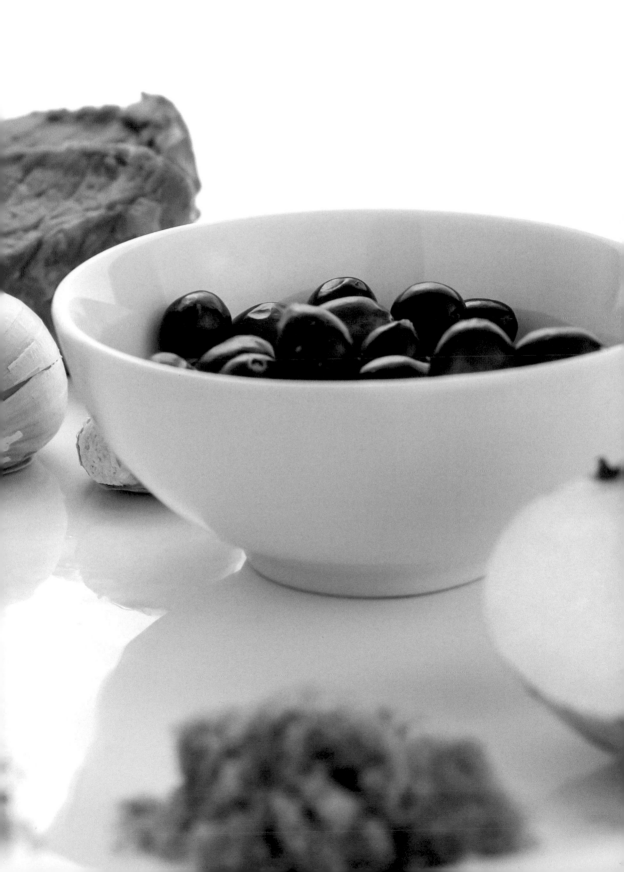

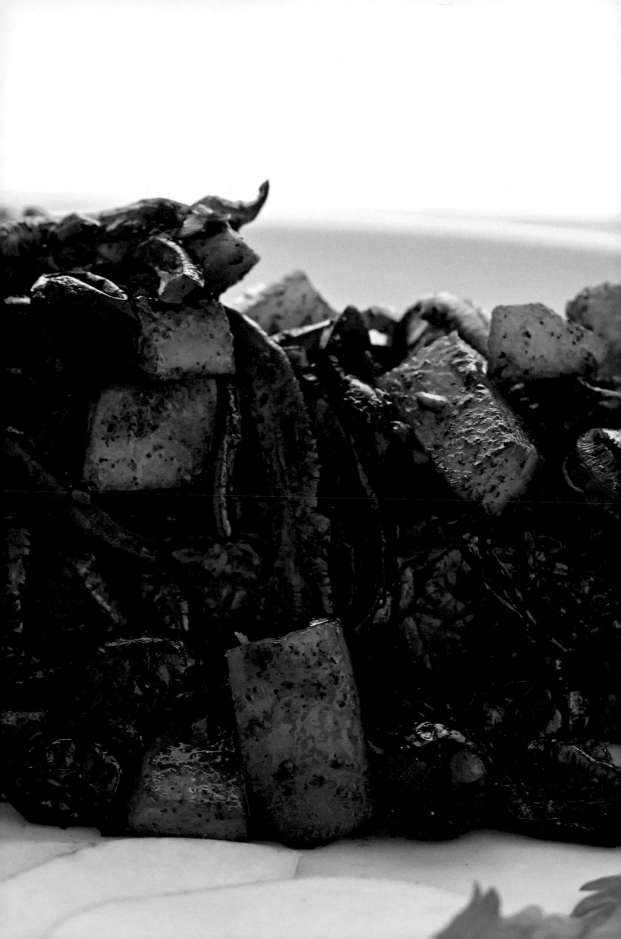

Servings	4
Prep Time	10 mins
Cooking Time	15 – 20 mins
PER SERVING	
Calories	237
Protein	25 grams
Carbohydrates	21 grams
Fat	5 grams

PEAR-CRANBERRY BEEF TENDERLOIN

4 beef tenderloin steaks, about 1 inch thick and trimmed of fat (4 ounces each)

1/2 large red onion, thinly sliced

2 cloves garlic, finely chopped

2 tablespoons dry red wine or grape juice

2 firm ripe pears, peeled and diced

1/2 cup fresh or frozen cranberries

2 tablespoons brown sugar

1/2 teaspoon pumpkin pie spice

> Spray a 12-inch skillet with cooking spray and place over medium-high heat. Add the onion, garlic, and wine. Sauté for about 3 minutes, until onion is tender but not brown.

> Add the pears, cranberries, brown sugar, and pumpkin pie spice. Reduce heat to medium-low. Simmer uncovered for about 10 minutes, stirring frequently, until the cranberries burst. Transfer chutney to bowl and set aside.

> Bring the heat back up to medium and add the beef to the skillet. Cook for about 4 minute on each side for medium doneness. Serve with the chutney.

SPICED PEPPER BEEF

Servings	4
Prep Time	5 mins
Cooking Time	15 – 20 mins

PER SERVING

Calories	165
Protein	24 grams
Carbohydrates	4 grams
Fat	5 grams

4 beef tenderloin steaks, about 1 inch thick and trimmed of fat (4 ounces each)

3 tablespoons low-carb ketchup

3 tablespoons water

3/4 teaspoon low-sodium soy sauce

1/2 medium green bell pepper, cut into thin strips

1 small onion, thinly sliced

coarsely ground black pepper, to taste

> Place beef between two pieces of parchment paper or plastic wrap, pound with a rolling pin or the flat side of a tenderizer to tenderize.

> In a small mixing bowl, combine the ketchup, water, and soy sauce and beat with a whisk until thoroughly blended.

> Coat a 10-inch skillet with cooking spray and place over medium-high heat. Cook beef in the skillet for 3 minutes, turning once. Add the bell peppers and onion and sauté. Add the ketchup mixture and reduce heat to low. Cover, let simmer for 12 minutes, or until the meat is desired doneness.

> Remove meat from pan and set aside. Bring the heat back up and add the ground pepper into the sauce left in the skillet, stir, then bring to a boil. Boil for 2 minutes, stirring frequently until sauce is slightly thickened. Spoon sauce over beef and serve.

BEEF TERIYAKI

4 sirloin steaks, trimmed of fat (6 ounces each)

1/3 cup low-sodium soy sauce

2 tablespoons molasses

2 teaspoons Dijon mustard

3 cloves garlic, minced

2 teaspoons ground ginger

salt and ground black pepper, to taste

Servings	4
Prep Time	5 mins (2 hrs marination)
Cooking Time	10 mins

PER SERVING

Calories	193
Protein	25 grams
Carbohydrates	11 grams
Fat	5 grams

> In a small mixing bowl, add the soy sauce, molasses, Dijon mustard, garlic, and ginger. Whisk together until mixed.

> Place the steaks in a large ziplock bag, sprinkle with salt and pepper, and pour in the marinade. Refrigerate for at least 2 hours, shaking occasionally.

> Heat a grill over high heat. Lightly coat with cooking spray and once the grill is hot, add the steak and grill 4 minutes undisturbed, flip and grill another 4 – 6 minutes, depending on preferred doneness.

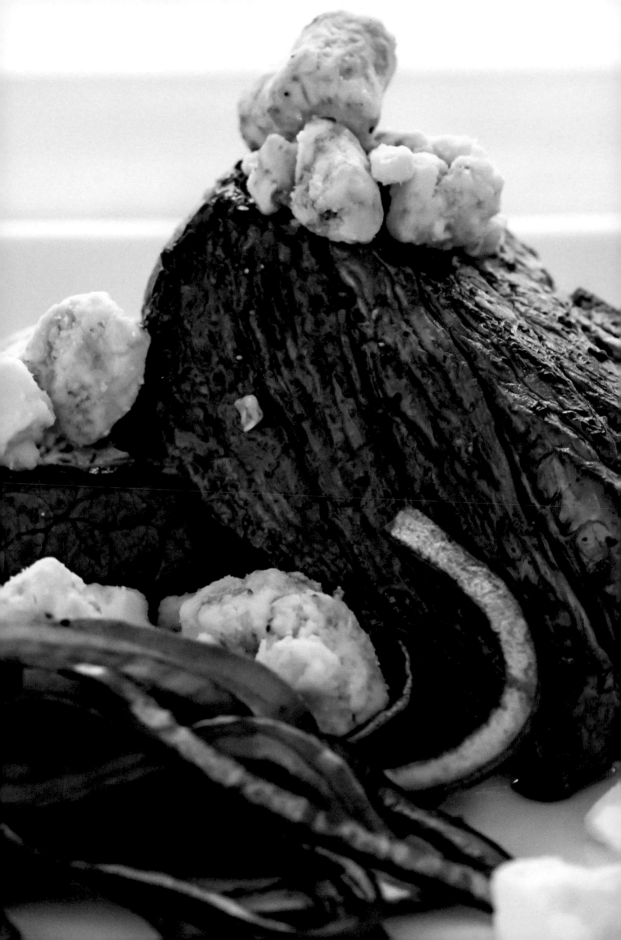

GORGONZOLA FILET WITH BALSAMIC ONIONS

Servings	4
Prep Time	2 – 3 mins
Cooking Time	15 – 20 mins
PER SERVING	
Calories	276
Protein	37 grams
Carbohydrates	7 grams
Fat	9 grams

4 extra-lean beef filets (6 ounces each)

3/4 teaspoon salt

3/4 teaspoon ground black pepper

1 large red onion, thinly sliced

1/4 cup balsamic vinegar

2 tablespoons crumbled Gorgonzola or blue cheese

> Preheat oven to 375°F. Rub filets evenly with 1/2 teaspoon each of the salt and pepper, set aside.

> Coat a baking sheet in cooking spray. Place onions in a mixing bowl, add the vinegar, remaining salt and pepper, toss to coat well. Transfer the onions to the baking sheet and spray with a light coating of cooking spray.

> Place onions in oven and bake for 20 minutes, or until onions are tender. Stir occasionally to prevent burning. Remove from oven and set aside.

> Meanwhile, coat a large skillet in cooking spray and place over medium-high heat. Add the filets and cook for 5 – 7 minutes on each side or until desired doneness. Top steaks evenly with cheese and onions.

SALISBURY STEAK

Servings	5
Prep Time	5 – 10 mins
Cooking Time	15 mins

PER SERVING

Calories	199
Protein	25 grams
Carbohydrates	12 grams
Fat	5 grams

1 pound extra-lean ground round or chuck

3 cups fresh mushrooms, sliced

1/4 cup plain bread crumbs

2 egg whites

1/4 cup skim milk

1/4 teaspoon dried thyme leaves

3 tablespoons low-carb ketchup

1 jar (12 ounces) fat-free beef gravy

> Finely chop 1 cup of the mushrooms and set the other 2 cups aside. In a medium-sized mixing bowl, combine the finely chopped mushrooms, ground beef, bread crumbs, egg whites, skim milk, thyme, and 1 tablespoon of the ketchup.

> Mix together very well. Shape the mixture into 5 oval patties, about 1/2 inch thick.

> Coat a 12-inch skillet in cooking spray and heat over medium-high heat. Add the patties and cook for about 2 – 3 minutes, flip and continue cooking for another 2 – 3 minutes, until brown.

> Add the remaining 2 cups of mushrooms, 2 tablespoons of ketchup, and gravy. Bring to a boil, then reduce heat to low. Cover and let simmer for 5 – 10 minutes, until patties reach desired doneness.

ADOBO SIRLOIN

4 extra-lean sirloin steaks (6 ounces each)

1 lime, juiced

1 tablespoon garlic, minced

1 teaspoon dried oregano

1 teaspoon ground cumin

2 tablespoons adobo sauce from canned peppers

2 tablespoons canned chipotle peppers in adobo sauce, finely chopped

salt and ground black pepper, to taste

Servings	4
Prep Time	5 mins (2 hrs for marination)
Cooking Time	10 – 15 mins

PER SERVING

Calories	213
Protein	37 grams
Carbohydrates	4 grams
Fat	7 grams

> In a small mixing bowl, combine the lime juice, garlic, oregano, cumin, and adobo sauce. Add chipotle peppers and mix well.

> Sprinkle some salt and pepper onto the meat, place into a ziplock bag and pour the adobo marinade over top. Place in refrigerator for at least 2 hours, shaking occasionally.

> Preheat a grill over high heat. Lightly coat the grill in cooking spray and once hot, place the steaks on the grill. Grill for 4 – 5 minutes on each side, until steaks reach desired doneness.

THAI BEEF KABOBS

1 pound beef tenderloin, trimmed of fat, cut into 2-inch cubes

2 tablespoons lemon juice

1 tablespoon low-sodium soy sauce

1 tablespoon garlic, minced

1 teaspoon red pepper flakes

1 teaspoon ground black pepper

Servings	4 (2 skewers per serving)
Prep Time	5 – 10 mins (2 hrs for marination)
Cooking Time	10 mins

PER SERVING

Calories	159
Protein	24 grams
Carbohydrates	2 grams
Fat	5 grams

> In a medium-sized mixing bowl, combine the lemon juice, soy sauce, garlic, red pepper flakes, and black pepper. Place the cubed beef into a ziplock bag and pour the marinade over. Place in refrigerator for at least 2 hours, shaking occasionally.

> Preheat the grill on high heat. Thread the beef evenly onto 8 skewers and place on the fully heated grill. Turn the steak every minute or two to brown all sides.

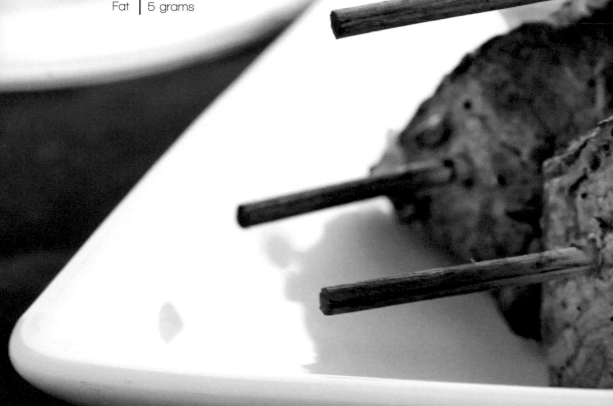

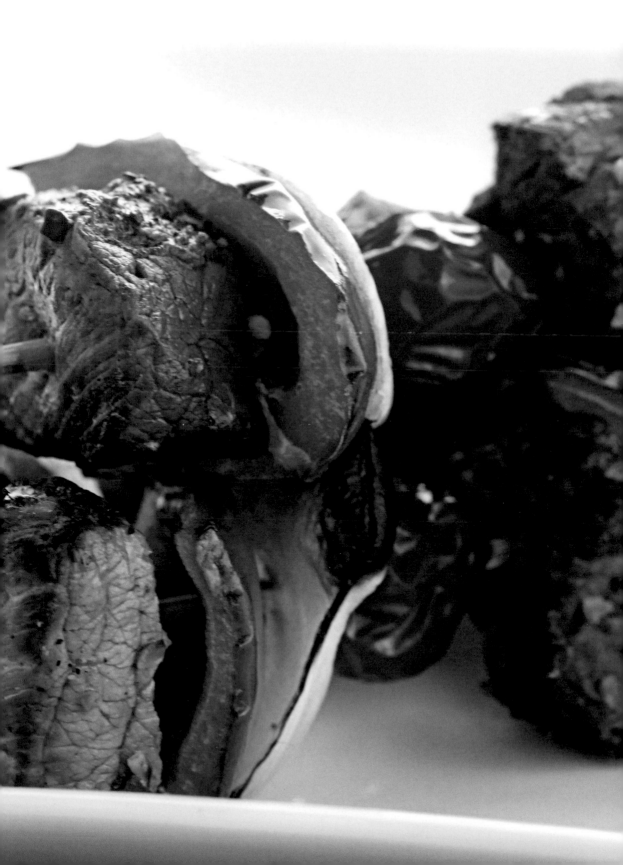

PORK

Pork is often criticized for its high fat content (especially ribs and bacon), but pork tenderloin is a good source of protein due to its high protein, low fat content, and versatility in terms of preparation. It's also a good source of B vitamins, niacin, and various minerals such as magnesium, iron, and zinc.

Whether dieting to lose weight or eating to gain muscle, pork can be a nice change from beef, chicken, and fish.

All of the recipes in this section of the book are suitable for both building muscle and losing weight due to being relatively low-calorie.

PLUM–MUSTARD PORK CHOPS

4 boneless pork chops, 1/2 inch thick, trimmed of fat (5 ounces each)

1/4 teaspoon salt

1/4 teaspoon ground black pepper

1/4 cup Chinese plum sauce or apricot jam

4 teaspoons yellow mustard

Servings	4
Prep Time	5 mins
Cooking Time	10 mins

PER SERVING

Calories	195
Protein	32 grams
Carbohydrates	7 grams
Fat	4 grams

> Spray a 10-inch nonstick skillet with cooking spray and place over medium-high heat. Rub the pork chops with the salt and pepper and place in skillet. Cook for 3 minutes on each side, until no longer pink in the center.

> In a small mixing bowl, mix the plum sauce and mustard. Spoon on top of the pork and serve.

CAJUN PORK CHOPS

4 boneless pork chops, 1/2 inch thick, trimmed of fat (5 ounces each)

2 teaspoons salt-free extra-spicy seasoning blend

1/2 medium onion, sliced

1 jalapeño peppers, seeded and finely chopped

1 can (14.5 ounces) diced tomatoes, undrained

Servings	4
Prep Time	10 mins
Cooking Time	15 – 20 mins

PER SERVING

Calories	194
Protein	33 grams
Carbohydrates	7 grams
Fat	4 grams

> Lay pork chops out and rub both sides with the spicy seasoning blend. Coat a 12-inch nonstick skillet in cooking spray and place over medium-high heat.

> Add the onion and jalapeño and sauté for 2 minutes, until slightly tender, push the mixture to one side of the skillet. On the other side, add the pork chops. Cook for 3 minutes, turning once to brown on both sides.

> Add the tomatoes and bring to a boil, reduce heat and cover. Cook for 6 – 8 minutes, or until pork chops are no longer pink in center.

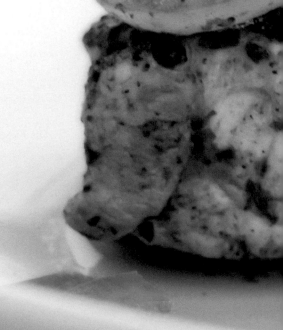

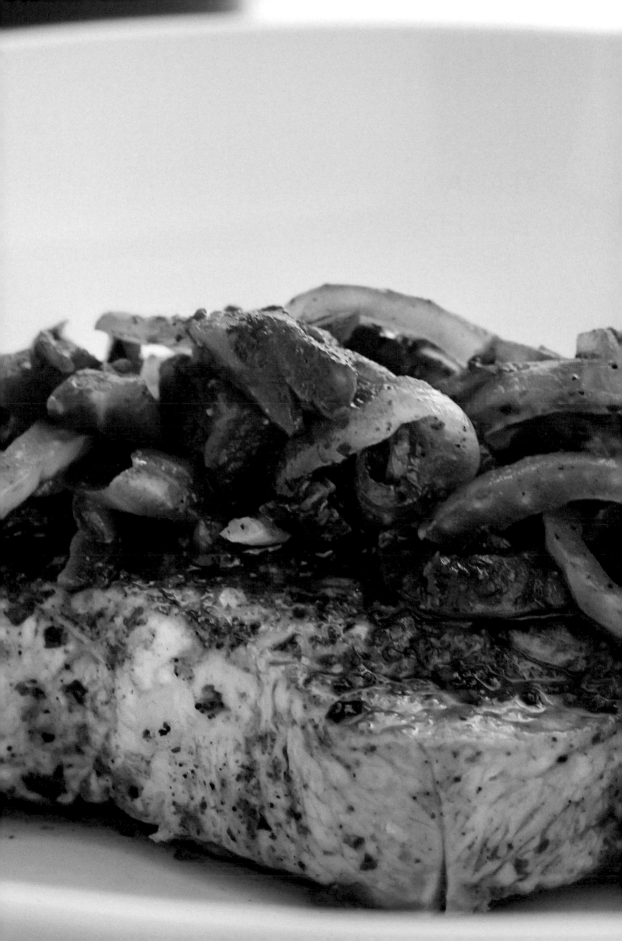

ITALIAN BAKED PORK

Servings	4
Prep Time	2 – 5 mins
Cooking Time	30 – 35 mins

PER SERVING

Calories	230
Protein	39 grams
Carbohydrates	0 grams
Fat	8 grams

2 pork tenderloins, trimmed of excess fat (12 ounces each)

1 tablespoon extra-virgin olive oil

1/2 teaspoon salt

1/4 teaspoon pepper

1/2 teaspoon fennel seed, crushed

1 clove garlic, finely chopped

> Preheat the oven to 375°F and coat a baking dish in cooking spray.

> In a small mixing bowl, combine the oil and seasoning and mash together with the back of a spoon until it becomes a paste. Place the pork in the baking dish and apply the paste evenly.

> Place the pork in the oven and roast for 25 – 35 minutes or until desired doneness. I personally like this dish to have a slight amount of pink in the center, which is about 160°F on a meat thermometer.

SLOW COOKED BONE-IN PORK CHOPS

Servings	4
Prep Time	5 mins
Cooking Time	4 – 5 hrs, or until tender

PER SERVING

Calories	359
Protein	32 grams
Carbohydrates	13 grams
Fat	20 grams

4 bone-in pork loin chops (8 ounces each)

1 teaspoon garlic powder

1/2 teaspoon salt

1/2 teaspoon ground pepper

2 cups low-carb ketchup

2 tablespoons brown sugar

> Rub the pork chops with garlic powder, salt, and pepper. Press into the meat.

> Coat a large skillet in cooking spray and place over medium-high heat. Place chops in skillet and brown on both sides.

> In a small mixing bowl, mix together the ketchup and brown sugar. Pour half the sauce into a 3-quart slow cooker. Place the pork chops on top of the sauce and pour the remaining sauce over top. Cover and cook over low heat for 4 – 5 hours, or until meat is desired doneness. Top with a little sauce.

BREADED PARMESAN PORK CHOPS

Servings	4
Prep Time	5 mins
Cooking Time	10 – 12 mins

PER SERVING

Calories	246
Protein	41 grams
Carbohydrates	9 grams
Fat	5 grams

4 boneless pork chops, 1/2 inch thick, trimmed of fat (6 ounces each)

1/4 cup skim milk

1/4 cup fat-free Parmesan cheese, grated

1/4 cup seasoned bread crumbs

1/4 teaspoon salt

1/8 teaspoon pepper

1/4 teaspoon garlic powder

> Preheat the oven to 375°F.

> Set up the milk in one bowl and the cheese, bread crumbs, salt, pepper, and garlic powder in another. Dunk the pork chops in the milk, then coat in the bread crumb mixture.

> Coat a baking sheet in cooking spray and transfer breaded chops to the sheet. Place in oven and bake for 9 – 11 minutes on each side, or until they reach desired level of doneness.

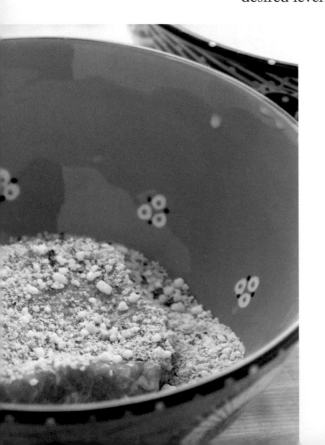

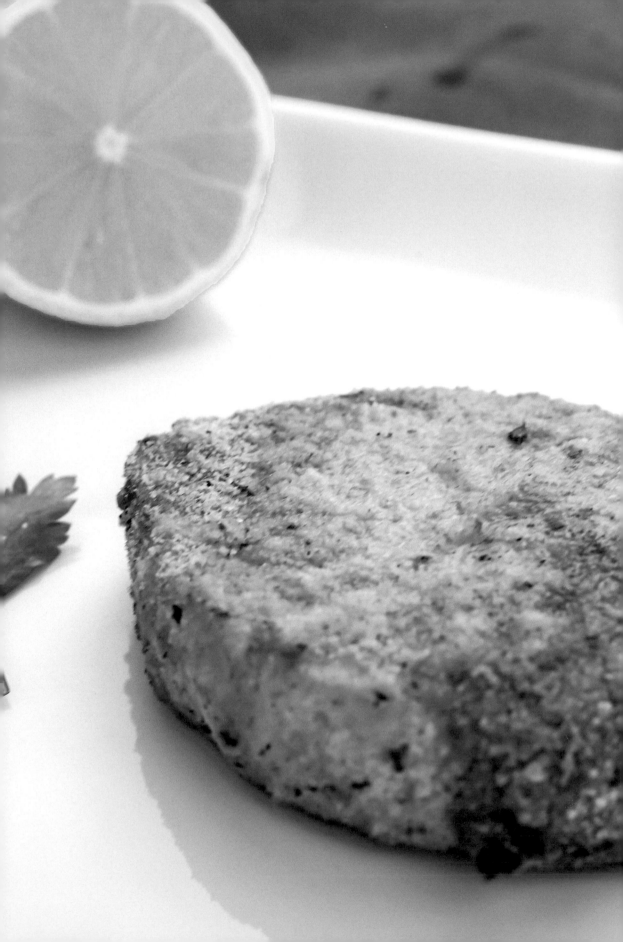

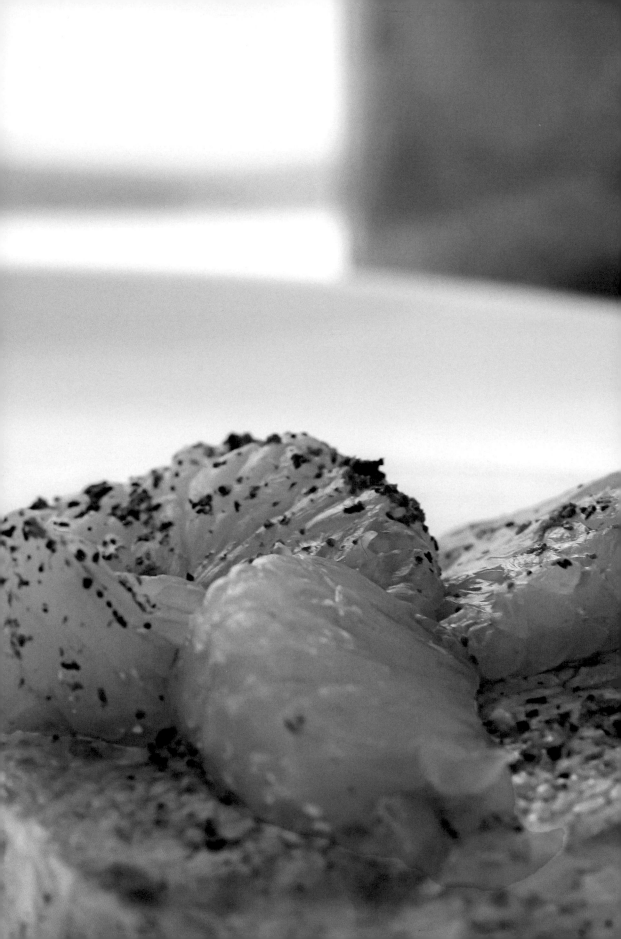

EASY ORANGE CHOPS

Servings	4
Prep Time	Under 5 mins
Cooking Time	20 – 25 mins
PER SERVING	
Calories	229
Protein	39 grams
Carbohydrates	7 grams
Fat	4 grams

4 boneless pork chops, 1/2 inch thick, trimmed of fat (6 ounces each)

salt and ground black pepper, to taste

1 can (11 ounces) mandarin oranges, drained

1/2 teaspoon ground cloves

> Sprinkle some salt and pepper over the chops, press into the meat. Coat a large skillet in cooking spray and place over medium-high heat.

> Place the chops in the pan and brown on both sides. Pour the oranges over top and sprinkle with the cloves. Cover with a tight fitting lid and reduce to a simmer. Cook for 20 – 25 minutes, or until meat reaches desired doneness.

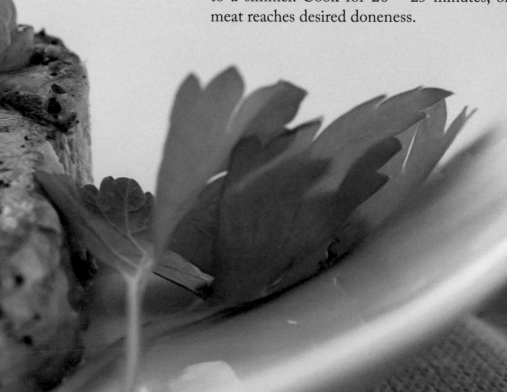

FISH & SEAFOOD

Fish is a terrific, healthy source of protein. It's high in omega-3 fatty acids, which can help fight inflammation, heart disease, and arthritis, and even improve brain function. Some of my favorite fish are tuna, halibut, tilapia, mahi-mahi, and salmon.

When buying fish, ensure it doesn't smell fishy. Fresh fish has a nice, salty sea smell, not a stinky odor, despite what the merchant may say.

A quick tip for cooking fish: Fish takes about 8 – 10 minutes to cook per inch of thickness, measured at its thickest part.

TUNA WITH FRESH PESTO

Servings	4
Prep Time	5 mins
Cooking Time	10 mins

PER SERVING

Calories	198
Protein	23 grams
Carbohydrates	3 grams
Fat	10 grams

4 tuna, swordfish, or other firm fish steaks, 3/4 inch thick (4 ounces each)

3 teaspoons extra-virgin olive oil

1/2 teaspoon salt

1 cup loosely packed fresh cilantro

1 cup loosely packed fresh Italian parsley (flat-leaf)

1/4 cup loosely packed fresh basil

4 medium scallions, sliced

1 clove garlic, cut in half

2 tablespoons lime juice

1/4 cup low-sodium chicken broth

1 tablespoon low-fat Parmesan cheese, grated

> Set oven to broil. Lay your tuna steaks out on a broiler dish and brush with 1 teaspoon of the extra-virgin olive oil.

> Place dish in the oven and broil with tops 4 inches from heat, for about 4 minutes. Remove from oven, turn over and sprinkle with 1/4 teaspoon of the salt, return to oven for another 4 – 5 minutes, until fish flakes easily with a fork and is slightly pink in the center.

> Meanwhile, combine the cilantro, parsley, basil, scallions, garlic, lime juice, 2 teaspoons oil, and 1/4 teaspoon salt in a food processor fitted with a metal blade attachment. Process for about 10 seconds, it should be finely chopped. With the food processor running, slowly add the chicken broth and process until almost smooth.

> Place in a mixing bowl and stir in the cheese, distribute evenly over each tuna steak.

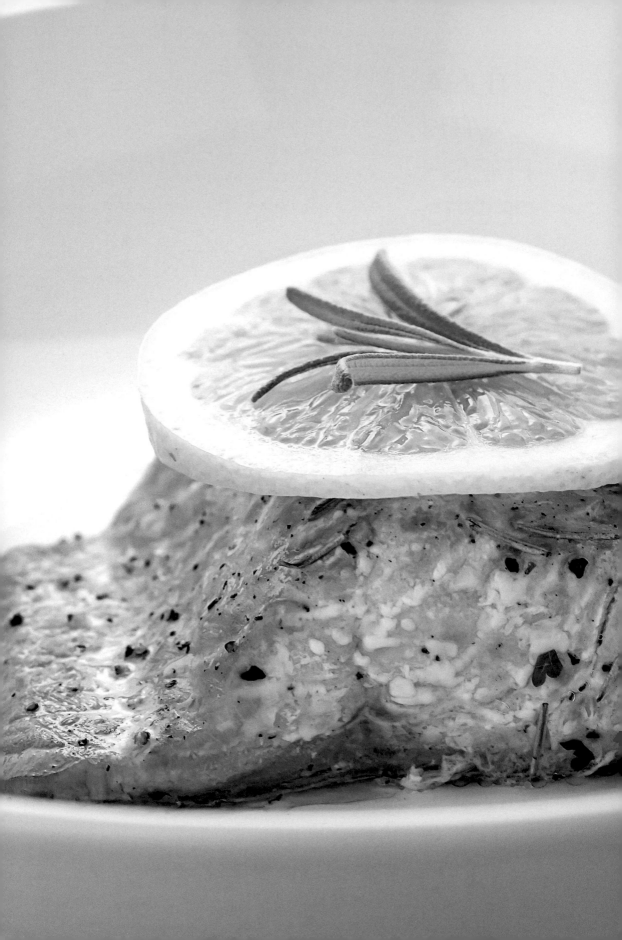

LEMON–ROSEMARY SALMON STEAKS

4 wild Atlantic salmon fillets (6 ounces each)

1 tablespoon lemon juice

1/2 teaspoon dried rosemary

1 tablespoon extra-virgin olive oil

salt and ground black pepper, to taste

Servings	4
Prep Time	15 mins marinating
Cooking Time	15 – 20 mins

PER SERVING

Calories	273
Protein	34 grams
Carbohydrates	0 grams
Fat	14 grams

> Preheat the oven to 350°F. Combine lemon juice, rosemary, and olive oil in a medium-sized baking dish.

> Season the salmon filets with salt and pepper. Add them to the baking dish and turn to coat. Allow to marinate for 10 – 15 minutes.

> Cover with foil and bake for about 20 minutes, or until fish flakes easily with a fork.

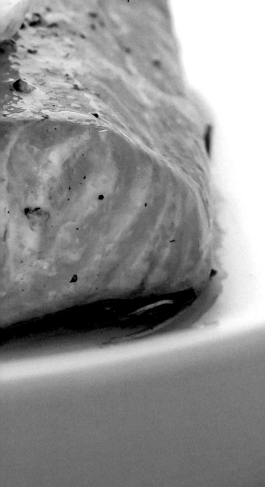

SUN-DRIED TOMATO SALMON FILETS

4 wild Atlantic salmon fillets, cooked (6 ounces each)

1/4 cup sun-dried tomatoes, sliced

1 teaspoon dried parsley flakes

2 garlic cloves, minced

salt and ground black pepper, to taste

1 tablespoon extra-virgin olive oil

Servings	4
Prep Time	5 mins
PER SERVING	
Calories	298
Protein	35 grams
Carbohydrates	2 gram
Fat	16 grams

> Pulse the sun-dried tomatoes, parsley, and garlic in a food processor until a paste forms. Add salt and pepper, and drizzle in the oil.

> To serve, top each cooked salmon filet with the sun-dried tomato mixture.

SALMON BURGERS

1 can (16 ounces) cooked salmon

1 egg

1/2 cup plain bread crumbs

1/2 small onion, diced

1 teaspoon Dijon mustard

1 tablespoon lemon juice

salt and ground black pepper, to taste

1 tablespoon extra-virgin olive oil

Servings	2
Prep Time	Under 5 mins
Cooking Time	5 mins
PER SERVING	
Calories	273
Protein	28 grams
Carbohydrates	11 grams
Fat	12 grams

> Drain salmon. In a medium bowl, combine with the rest of the ingredients, except oil. Form into 4 patties.

> Heat oil in a large skillet over medium-high heat. Add salmon burgers and cook for 1 – 2 minutes per side, or until browned.

Servings	4
Prep Time	5 – 10 mins
Cooking Time	10 mins
PER SERVING	
Calories	225
Protein	25 grams
Carbohydrates	10 grams
Fat	10 grams

GRAHAM-COATED TILAPIA

4 fresh tilapia fillets, about 3/4 inch thick (4 ounces each)

1/2 cup plain graham cracker crumbs

1 teaspoon lemon zest

1/4 teaspoon salt

1/4 teaspoon ground black pepper

1/4 cup skim milk

1 tablespoon canola oil

2 tablespoons toasted pecans, chopped

> Position the oven rack to slightly above the middle point. Heat oven to 500°F. Cut the fish crosswise into 2-inch-wide pieces. In a small mixing bowl, add the graham cracker, lemon zest, salt, and pepper. Place the skim milk in a separate mixing bowl.

> Dunk the fish in the milk, then lightly coat with the cracker mix and transfer to a 13 x 9 inch baking dish. Drizzle the oil and pecans over the fish and place in oven. Bake for about 10 minutes, or until fish flakes easily with a fork.

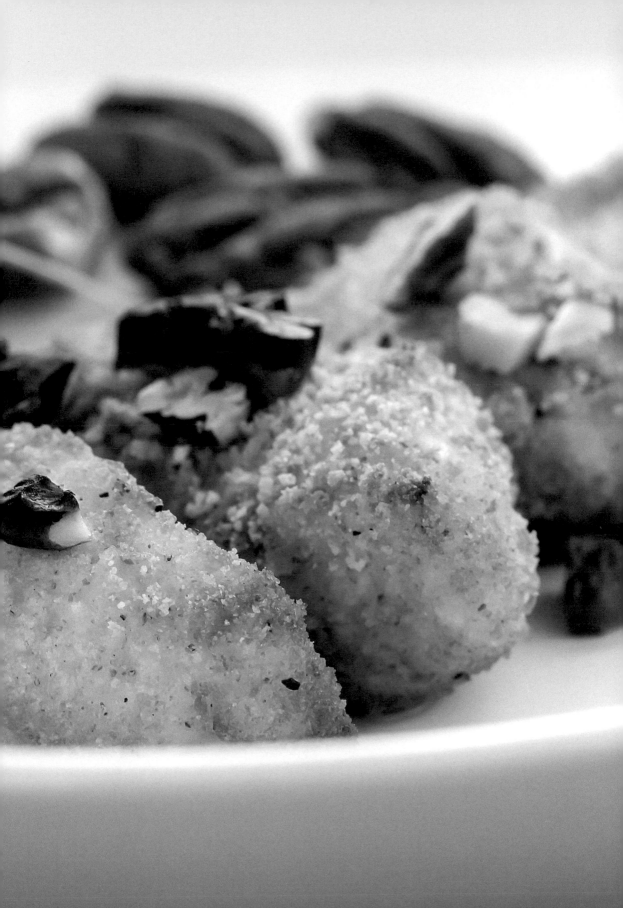

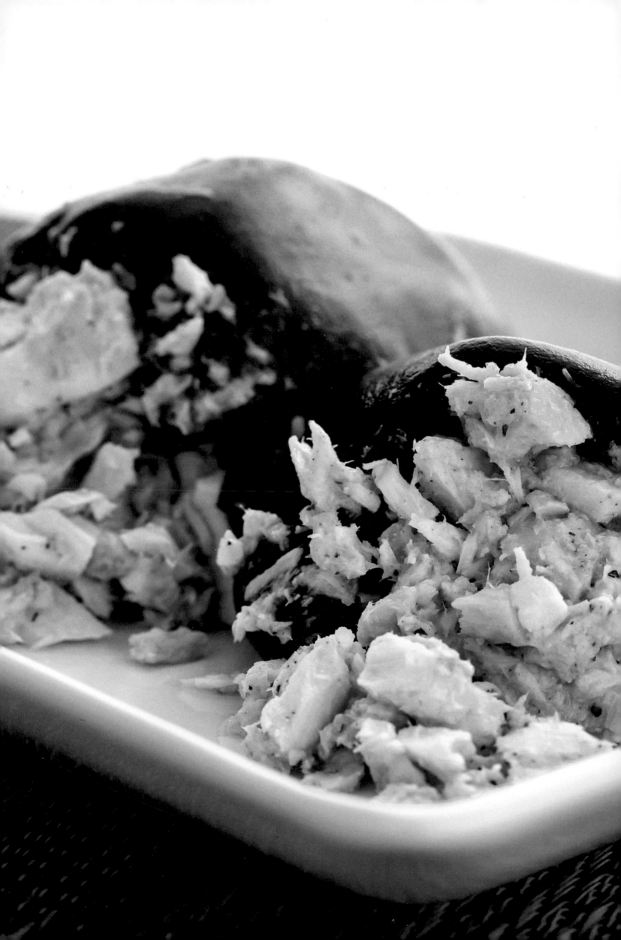

TUNA SALAD STUFFED PEPPERS

Servings	4 (3 peppers per serving)
Prep Time	5 – 10 mins

PER SERVING

Calories	152
Protein	22 grams
Carbohydrates	6 grams
Fat	4 grams

2 cans (6 ounces each) chunk tuna in oil, drained

1/2 teaspoon smoked paprika

1/2 teaspoon lemon zest

1 tablespoon lemon juice

1 tablespoon extra-virgin olive oil

salt and ground black pepper, to taste

1 jar (12) whole piquillo peppers

12 medium-sized whole basil leaves

> In a medium-sized mixing bowl, add the tuna and separate. Stir in the paprika, lemon zest, lemon juice, oil, salt, and pepper, and mix well.

> Dry the peppers and carefully split them open, rolling them out flat. Remove the seeds, then add a whole basil leaf, top with the tuna mixture and roll to close.

SAVORY SOY AND WHITE WINE HALIBUT

4 halibut filets (6 ounces each)

2 tablespoons extra-virgin olive oil

2 tablespoons low-sodium soy sauce

2 tablespoons lemon juice

2 tablespoons white wine

2 cloves garlic, minced

2 (quarter-sized) pieces fresh ginger, peeled and minced

salt and ground black pepper, to taste

3 medium leeks (white part only), thinly sliced

2 red bell peppers, seeded and thinly sliced

Servings	4
Prep Time	10 mins & 1 hr marination
Cooking Time	30 mins

PER SERVING

Calories	365
Protein	47 grams
Carbohydrates	16 grams
Fat	12 grams

> In a medium-sized mixing bowl, add the olive oil, soy sauce, lemon juice, white wine, garlic, ginger, salt, and pepper, and mix well. Put the halibut in a ziplock bag and pour the marinade over top. Place in refrigerator for at least 1 hour, shaking occasionally.

> Preheat the broiler. Remove the fish from the marinade and set aside. Place a large skillet over medium heat and pour in the marinade. Add the leeks and red pepper and cook for 15 minutes, or until tender.

> Meanwhile, place the fish on a baking pan and under the broiler, 4 – 6 inches from the heat. Cook 4 – 5 minutes, flip and cook another 4 minutes, or until flesh is opaque through and flakes easily. Top with vegetables and sauce.

CREAMY SCALLOP FETTUCCINE

Servings	5 (1 1/2 cups per serving)
Prep Time	10 – 15 mins
Cooking Time	20 mins

PER SERVING

Calories	361
Protein	32 grams
Carbohydrates	47 grams
Fat	4 grams

1 pound large sea scallops

8 ounces whole grain fettuccine

1 bottle (8 ounces) clam juice (get lowest sodium you can find)

1 cup skim milk

3 tablespoons cornstarch

salt and ground black pepper, to taste

3 cups frozen peas, thawed

1/2 cup low-fat Parmesan cheese, grated

1/3 cup chives, chopped

1/2 teaspoon lemon zest

1 teaspoon lemon juice

> Cook pasta according to package directions.

> Meanwhile, dry the scallops with a paper towel and sprinkle with salt. Coat a large nonstick skillet with cooking spray and place over medium-high heat. Add the scallops and cook until golden brown, about 2 – 3 minutes per side. Remove from pan and set aside.

> Add the clam juice to the pan. In a medium-sized mixing bowl, add the milk, cornstarch, salt, and pepper, and whisk until smooth. Pour the milk mixture into the pan and whisk with the clam juice. Once the mixture is simmering, stir constantly until sauce has thickened, about 1 – 2 minutes.

> Place the scallops and peas into the clam sauce and bring to a simmer. Add the fettuccine, chives, lemon zest, lemon juice, and most of the Parmesan, and mix together well. Remove from heat and top with a little extra cheese.

LEMON-GARLIC SHRIMP

Servings	4
Prep Time	10 mins
Cooking Time	10 – 15 mins

PER SERVING

Calories	205
Protein	30 grams
Carbohydrates	15 grams
Fat	4 grams

1 pound raw shrimp

2 red bell peppers, seeded and diced

2 pounds asparagus, cut into 1-inch pieces

2 teaspoons lemon zest

1/2 teaspoon salt

2 teaspoons extra-virgin olive oil

5 cloves garlic, minced

1 cup low-sodium chicken broth

1 teaspoon cornstarch

2 tablespoons lemon juice

2 tablespoons fresh parsley, chopped

> Coat a large nonstick skillet with cooking spray and place over medium-high heat. Add the bell peppers, asparagus, lemon zest, and 1/4 teaspoon of the salt. Sauté until vegetables begin to soften, about 6 minutes. Transfer vegetables to a bowl, cover, and set aside.

> Add the oil and garlic to the pan and sauté for 30 seconds. Stir in the shrimp. In a small bowl, add the broth and cornstarch and whisk to combine. Pour in the broth mixture and remaining 1/4 teaspoon of salt and stir.

> Cook, stirring frequently, until the sauce thickens and the shrimp are pink and cooked through, about 2 – 3 minutes. Remove from the heat, add the lemon juice and parsley, mix together, and serve the shrimp over the vegetables.

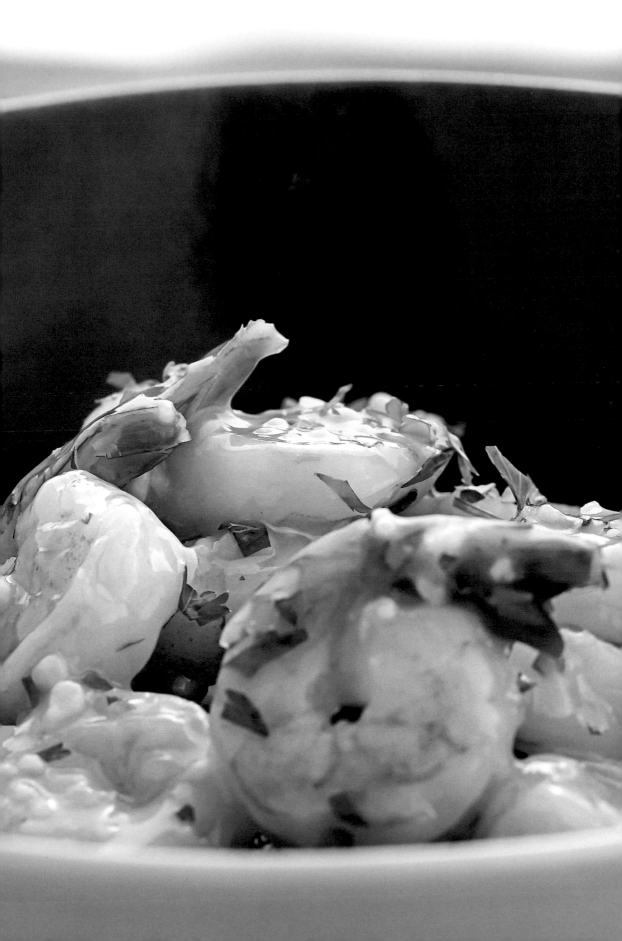

SEARED WASABI TUNA

4 tuna steaks, about 3/4 inch thick (6 ounces each)

1 3/4 cup water

3 large ears of corn, shucked and kernels removed (about 2 cups)

1 teaspoon wasabi paste

salt, to taste

Servings	4
Prep Time	Under 5 mins
Cooking Time	35 – 40 mins

PER SERVING

Calories	250
Protein	43 grams
Carbohydrates	15 grams
Fat	3 grams

> In a small saucepan, add 1 3/4 cups water, 1 1/2 cups of corn, and salt. Bring to a boil over medium-high heat, then reduce heat and simmer until corn is very soft, about 20 minutes. Transfer cooked corn to a blender and blend until smooth. Pour into a small mixing bowl, add the wasabi paste, and mix thoroughly.

> Place the small saucepan back over medium heat and add the remaining 1/2 cup of corn and just enough water to cover. Cook for 10 minutes, or until corn is soft.

> Meanwhile, add salt to both sides of the tuna steaks and rub into meat. Coat a large nonstick skillet with cooking spray and place over medium-high heat. Once pan is hot, add the tuna and sear each side, about 3 minutes.

> Drain the corn, plate the fish and top with corn and wasabi sauce.

5 FAST & SIMPLE CANNED TUNA RECIPES

Canned tuna is a great fast food because it's high in protein, low in fat, and can be quickly prepared in many ways. Each of these recipes can be prepared in less than 15 minutes.

Below are five different ways to make quick and tasty canned tuna snacks. I recommend that you stick to the lowest-sodium brands packed in water.

TUNA SALAD STUFFED PITA

3 ounces canned tuna (drained)

1 hardboiled egg white

2 tablespoons diced celery

2 tablespoons raisins

1 tablespoon diced scallion

2 teaspoons low-fat mayonnaise

1/2 teaspoon Dijon mustard

2 tablespoons diced pineapple

1 whole grain pita

In a medium-sized mixing bowl, add all of the ingredients except the pita. Mix until well combined, divide into 2 equal portions. Cut the pita in half, stuff each half with 1 portion of the tuna salad.

Servings	2
Calories	184
Protein	16 grams
Carbohydrates	28 grams
Fat	2 grams

TUNA MELT

3 ounces canned tuna (drained)

1 teaspoon low-fat mayonnaise

dash of hot sauce

1/2 teaspoon lemon juice

2 slices whole grain bread

2 slices tomato

deli slice of low-fat cheddar cheese

salt and ground black pepper, to taste

In a medium-sized mixing bowl, add the tuna, mayo, hot sauce, lemon juice, salt, and pepper. Mix until well combined. Place on whole grain bread, top with tomato slices, cheese, and remaining slice of bread. Melt the cheese in an oven or toaster oven.

Servings	1
Calories	340
Protein	38 grams
Carbohydrates	32 grams
Fat	7 grams

SCHOOLYARD TUNA

3 ounces canned tuna (drained)

1/4 cup low-fat cottage cheese

3 tablespoons sliced almonds

3 tablespoons raisins

2 tablespoons carrots, shredded

In a medium-sized mixing bowl, add all of the ingredients and mix until well combined.

Servings	1
Calories	349
Protein	34 grams
Carbohydrates	34 grams
Fat	7 grams

TUNA WITH PICO DE GALLO

6 ounces canned tuna (drained)

2 diced Roma tomatoes

1/4 cup chopped fresh cilantro

2 tablespoons lime juice

1/4 cup diced red onion

1 diced small serrano chili

4 pieces toasted whole grain bread

1/2 teaspoon salt

In a medium-sized mixing bowl, add all of the ingredients except the bread. Mix until well combined, divide into 4 equal portions, and serve with piece of toasted whole grain bread.

Servings	4
Calories	150
Protein	16 grams
Carbohydrates	17 grams
Fat	2 grams

SPICY TUNA

3 ounces canned tuna (drained)

1 tablespoon diced pickled jalapeños

1 teaspoon hot sauce

4 tablespoons diced tomatoes

1/8 teaspoon cayenne pepper

salt and ground black pepper, to taste

In a medium-sized mixing bowl, add all of the ingredients and mix until well combined.

Servings	1
Calories	117
Protein	22 grams
Carbohydrates	4 grams
Fat	1 gram

PASTA & GRAINS

Carbohydrates are a vital source of energy for your body. They provide fuel in the form of glucose and glycogen and are the macronutrient that you manipulate most when trying to gain muscle or lose fat. When you're eating to gain muscle, the abundance of carbs in your diet not only increases your strength and endurance in the gym, but also gives you an overall sense of satiety and well-being. When you're eating to lose fat, your drastically lowered carb intake not only leads to dropped pounds, but also gives you that dry, hard look.

A good source of slow-burning, low-fat carbohydrates are whole grains such as wheat, brown rice, quinoa, oats, and barley. What are whole grains, exactly? They're grains that contain all the essential parts and naturally occurring nutrients of the entire grain seed. If the grain has been processed (cracked, crushed, rolled, chopped up, or cooked) and still has 100% of the original kernel, it's still a whole-grain product.

In contrast to whole grains are refined grains, which are grains that have been considerably modified from their natural state. Modifications include processes that remove essential parts of the grain, bleaching, and mixing back in a fraction of the nutrients removed.

So, stick to the whole grains and reap their many benefits, such as reduced risk of stroke, diabetes, and heart disease, healthier blood pressure levels, reduction of inflammation, and more.

As you'll see, the pasta recipes in this section always have some form of protein added because one serving of whole-grain pasta has only about 7 grams of protein.

As a note, the pasta measurements given are the dry weight. You'll need a scale to measure them exactly.

Also, I recommend lightly salting the pasta water and <u>not</u> adding oil to the water. Doing so actually makes it harder for the sauce to stick to the pasta.

CHICKEN CACCIATORE

Servings	4
Prep Time	5 mins
Cooking Time	40 – 45 mins
PER SERVING	
Calories	454
Protein	45 grams
Carbohydrates	48 grams
Fat	7 grams

6 ounces quinoa rotelle pasta

4 boneless, skinless chicken breasts (6 ounces), rinsed, dried, trimmed of fat, cut into strips

1 tablespoon vegetable oil

1/2 medium onion, chopped

1/2 cup fresh mushrooms, thinly sliced

1 clove garlic, minced

1 can (28 ounces) of plum tomatoes, with juice

1/2 cup dry red wine

1 teaspoon dried oregano

1 bay leaf

1/2 cup fresh parsley, chopped

> Heat the oil in a large, deep skillet over medium-high heat. Add the chicken and brown on both sides. Add the onions, mushrooms, and garlic and sauté until vegetables are tender.

> Add the tomatoes, wine, oregano, and bay leaf and reduce heat to medium-low. Cover and simmer for 30 – 35 minutes, or until chicken is cooked through and sauce has thickened. Stir occasionally.

> Meanwhile, cook the pasta according to package directions.

> Add the cooked pasta and 1/4 cup of the pasta water to the chicken, cook for 1 – 2 minutes, mixing well so the sauce sticks to the pasta. Remove bay leaf and top with fresh parsley.

CHICKEN PESTO PASTA

4 ounces whole grain ziti

1 boneless, skinless chicken breast (6 ounces), rinsed, dried, trimmed of fat, cut into small cubes

25 fresh basil leaves, finely chopped

1 teaspoon garlic, minced

1 tablespoon warm water

2 tablespoons crushed pine nuts

1 tablespoon extra-virgin olive oil

salt and ground black pepper, to taste

2 tablespoons Parmesan cheese, grated

Servings	2
Prep Time	5 mins
Cooking Time	20 mins
PER SERVING	
Calories	446
Protein	32 grams
Carbohydrates	43 grams
Fat	16 grams

> Bring a pot of lightly salted water to a boil, cook the pasta according to the package directions.

> In a large bowl, mix the basil, garlic, water, pine nuts, and oil.

> Turn on the stove to medium heat and coat your pan or skillet with cooking spray.

> Begin to cook the chicken in the pan. Once almost cooked, reduce the heat and stir in your salt, pepper, pesto, and Parmesan. Cook until chicken is no longer pink on inside, stir into cooked pasta.

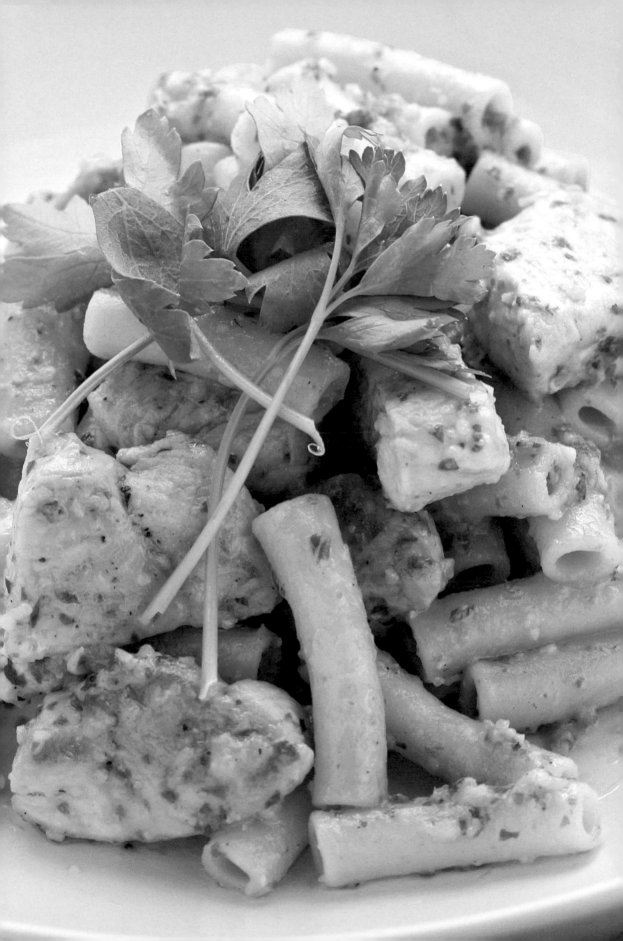

CHICKEN FETTUCCINE WITH MUSHROOMS

Servings	4
Prep Time	5 – 10 mins
Cooking Time	15 – 20 mins

PER SERVING

Calories	403
Protein	34 grams
Carbohydrates	38 grams
Fat	12 grams

8 ounces whole grain fettuccine

2 boneless, skinless chicken breasts (6 ounces each), rinsed, dried, trimmed of fat, cut into strips

2 tablespoons extra-virgin olive oil

3 cloves garlic, minced

2 ounces (around 1 to 1 1/2 cups) shiitake mushrooms, stemmed and sliced

2 tablespoons lemon juice

2 teaspoons lemon zest

salt and ground black pepper, to taste

1/2 cup Parmesan cheese, grated

1/2 cup fresh basil, chopped

> Cook pasta according to package directions. When you drain the pasta, save 1/2 cup of the pasta water.

> Meanwhile, heat the oil in a large nonstick skillet over medium heat. Add the sliced chicken and cook for 3 – 4 minutes, add the garlic and mushrooms. Cook, stirring occasionally for 4 – 5 minutes or until the mushrooms are nice and tender. Stir in the lemon juice, lemon zest, salt, and pepper and remove from the heat.

> Add the pasta, 1/2 cup of pasta water, Parmesan, and basil to the skillet and toss.

PASTA SALAD WITH CHICKEN

Servings	6
Prep Time	10 mins
Cooking Time	20 – 25 mins

PER SERVING

Calories	381
Protein	27 grams
Carbohydrates	41 grams
Fat	12 grams

8 ounces whole grain bow-tie pasta

3 cups (about 3 breasts) cooked chicken breast, shredded

1 can (8 ounces) chickpeas, drained and rinsed

1 can (2.25 ounces) sliced black olives, drained

2 sticks of celery, chopped

2 cucumbers, peeled and cut into chunks

1/2 cup carrots, shredded

1/2 cup sweet onion, chopped

2 tablespoons Parmesan cheese, shredded

3 tablespoons extra-virgin olive oil

1/2 cup red wine vinegar

1/2 teaspoon Worcestershire sauce

1/2 teaspoon spicy brown mustard

1/2 teaspoon garlic, minced

2 tablespoons fresh Italian parsley, chopped

1 tablespoon fresh basil, chopped or 1 teaspoon dried basil

1/4 teaspoon ground black pepper

> Cook the pasta according to the package directions; drain. Run pasta under cold water for about 30 seconds or until completely cool, then transfer to a large mixing bowl.

> Add the remaining ingredients and mix thoroughly.

> Cover the bowl and place in the refrigerator overnight, or for at least 4 hours. Mix prior to serving.

BEEF LASAGNA

Servings	4
Prep Time	10 mins
Cooking Time	50 mins – 1 hr

PER SERVING

Calories	279
Protein	24 grams
Carbohydrates	34 grams
Fat	4 grams

6 no-boil lasagna noodles

1/2 pound extra-lean ground round

1 teaspoon extra-virgin olive oil

1/2 small yellow onion, chopped

1/2 teaspoon dried oregano

pinch of ground black pepper

2 cups low-sodium tomato sauce

1 cup fat-free ricotta cheese

1 tablespoon Parmesan cheese, grated

1 zucchini, thinly sliced

> Preheat the oven to 350°F.

> Heat oil in a large nonstick skillet over medium-high heat. Add the ground beef, onion, oregano, and pepper. Stir while breaking apart the beef, for about 6 – 8 minutes, or until the beef is fully cooked. Stir in the tomato sauce and bring to a boil, then remove from the heat.

> In a bowl, mix the ricotta and Parmesan.

> Now, to build the lasagna, take a 9 x 5 inch baking dish and begin by layering 1/2 cup of the sauce, 2 of the noodles, 1/2 cup of the cheese mix, another 1/2 cup of the sauce, and 1/2 of the zucchini. Add the next 2 noodles and repeat 1/2 cup of cheese, 1/2 cup of sauce, and 1/2 of the zucchini. Finish by topping the zucchini with the remaining 1/2 cup of sauce and 2 noodles.

> Cover the dish with foil and bake in the oven for 30 minutes.

> Remove the foil, then bake for 15 minutes longer. Remove from the oven and let sit for at least 10 minutes before serving.

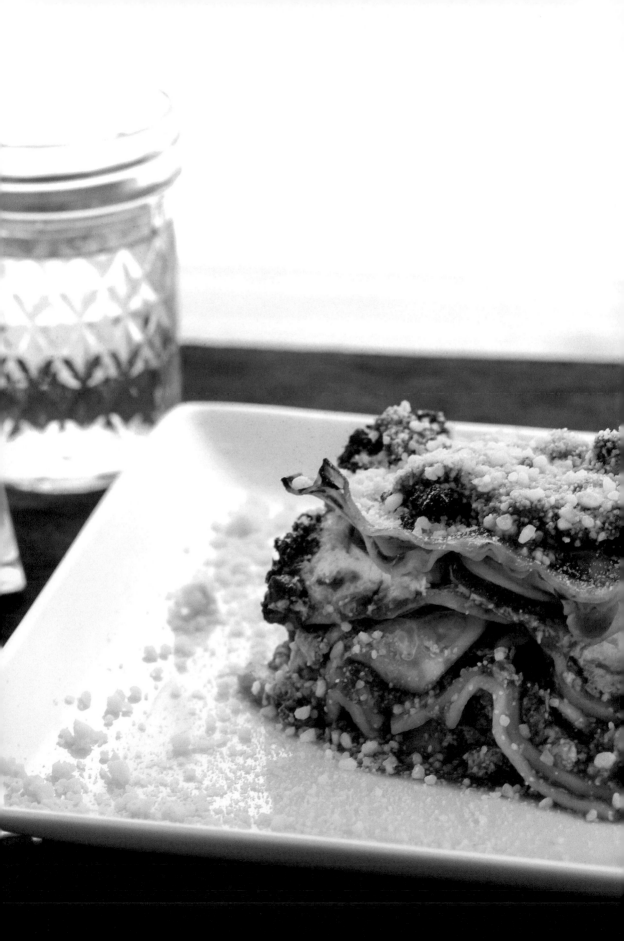

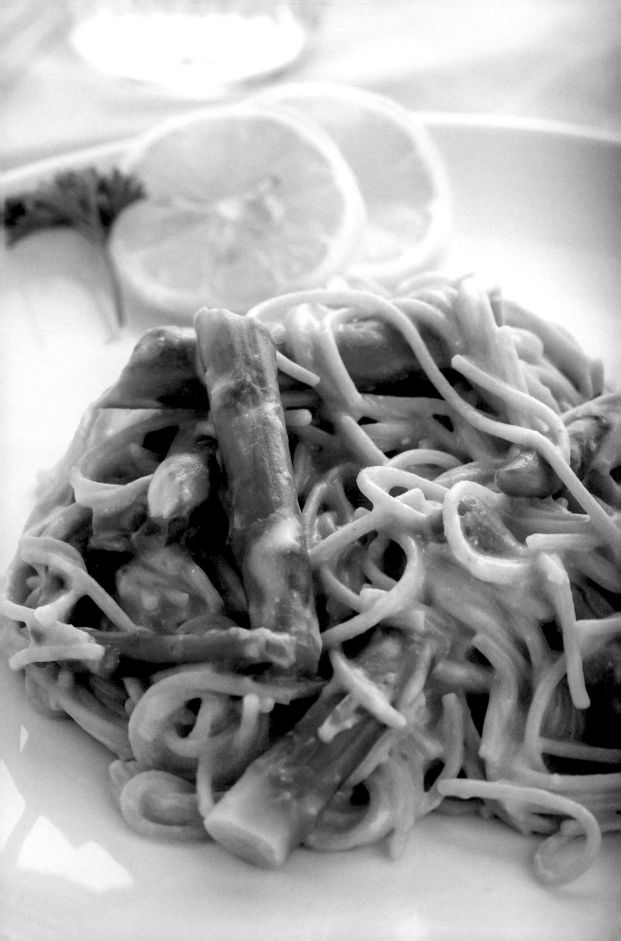

ASPARAGUS AND GOAT CHEESE PASTA

Servings	4
Prep Time	5 mins
Cooking Time	20 mins
PER SERVING	
Calories	389
Protein	20 grams
Carbohydrates	50 grams
Fat	13 grams

8 ounces whole grain thin spaghetti

1 pound asparagus, with bottoms cut off

1 tablespoon unsalted butter

2 tablespoons all-purpose flour

1 can (14 ounce) low-sodium chicken broth

4 ounces goat cheese

1 teaspoon lemon zest

pinch of ground black pepper

1/2 cup Parmesan cheese, grated

> Bring a large pot of lightly salted water to a boil and add the noodles, cook to package instructions.

> Meanwhile, heat a large pan of lightly salted water to boiling over high heat. Add the asparagus and blanch in the boiling water for 3 minutes, or until they turn bright green. Remove and rinse under cold water to stop the cooking.

> Heat a saucepan over medium-high heat, add the butter. Once the butter is melted whisk in the flour. Add the broth and cook for 2 minutes, stirring constantly, until the sauce thickens. Mix in the goat cheese and lemon zest.

> Add the spaghetti and asparagus to the pan and toss, covering the pasta in sauce. Serve with pepper and the Parmesan.

PORK TENDERLOIN STIR-FRY

Servings	4
Prep Time	5 mins
Cooking Time	15 mins

PER SERVING

Calories	461
Protein	36 grams
Carbohydrates	62 grams
Fat	8 grams

8 ounces rice noodles

1 pound pork tenderloin, trimmed of fat

1/3 cup water

1/4 cup Shao Hsing rice wine or dry sherry

2 tablespoons low-sodium soy sauce

2 teaspoons cornstarch

1 tablespoon peanut oil or canola oil

1 medium onion, thinly sliced

1 pound bok choy (about 1 medium head), trimmed and cut into long, thin strips

1 tablespoon garlic, minced

1 tablespoon chili-garlic sauce

> Bring a large pot of lightly salted water to a boil and add noodles, cook according to package instructions. Drain, quickly rinse with cold water to stop from further cooking.

> While the pasta is boiling, slice the pork into thin rounds, then cut each round into matchsticks.

> In a small bowl whisk the water, rice wine (or sherry), soy sauce, and cornstarch.

> Heat the oil in a Dutch oven over medium heat. Add the onion and cook for 2 – 3 minutes. Once the onions are softened, add the bok choy and cook, stirring occasionally until it begins to soften, about 5 minutes. Add the pork, garlic, and chili-garlic sauce. Stir occasionally until the pork is just cooked through, about 2 – 3 minutes.

> Take your cornstarch mixture and give it a quick whisk, then add to the Dutch oven and bring to a boil. Stir frequently for 2 – 4 minutes until the sauce has thickened. Serve on top of the noodles.

SALADS

The Shredded Chef is all about eating healthy, high-quality proteins, carbs, and fats to maximize muscle growth and fat loss. Whole grains and animal proteins are a vital part of this, as are plant foods. Fruit and vegetables provide essential vitamins and minerals that support many physiological processes connected not only with building muscle and losing fat, but also with general health and vitality.

The one pitfall of salads is *dressing*. Pretty much every dressing you could buy in your local grocery store is full of sodium, unhealthy fats, and chemical additives. That's why I recommend making your own dressings from high-quality ingredients.

A little trick I learned for eating less dressing (important when dieting to lose weight) is to do the following: instead of spooning a bunch of dressing over your salad, keep it on the side. Dip your fork in it before each bite, and drizzle it over a few bites' worth of salad. You won't feel cheated in terms of taste and will be surprised at how much less dressing you use by doing this.

Delicious salads are a great way to get in some of your daily servings of fruit and vegetables. I eat a salad almost every day, regardless of whether I'm eating to gain muscle or lose fat.

This section starts with some recipes for a few healthy salad dressings (in case you don't want to make one of the full-blown recipes given) and then gets into some full-salad recipes.

RED WINE VINAIGRETTE DRESSING

2 tablespoons extra-virgin olive oil

2 tablespoons red wine vinegar

1/2 teaspoon Dijon mustard

1/4 teaspoon dried thyme

1/4 teaspoon minced garlic

pinch of ground black pepper

> Mix all the ingredients in a bowl (how's that for simple?).

Servings	2
Calories	124
Protein	0 grams
Carbohydrates	0 grams
Fat	14 grams

BALSAMIC VINAIGRETTE

2 tablespoons extra-virgin olive oil

2 tablespoons balsamic vinegar

1/2 teaspoon fresh basil, chopped

1/2 teaspoon honey mustard (use the lowest sodium one you can find)

1/4 teaspoon minced garlic

pinch of ground black pepper

> Mix all the ingredients in a bowl.

Servings	2
Calories	133
Protein	0 grams
Carbohydrates	2 grams
Fat	14 grams

CREAMY WHITE VINEGAR DRESSING

1/4 cup fat-free plain yogurt

1 tablespoon fat-free sour cream

1 tablespoon fresh cilantro, chopped

1 teaspoon white vinegar

1/4 teaspoon minced garlic

pinch of ground black or white pepper

> Mix all the ingredients in a bowl.

Servings	4
Calories	11
Protein	1 gram
Carbohydrates	2 grams
Fat	0 grams

STEAK AND SWEET POTATO SALAD

1 filet mignon, about 1 inch thick (8 ounces)

1/2 tablespoon ground black pepper

1 large sweet potato

4 medium white button mushrooms, stems trimmed and sliced

2 scallions, thinly sliced

2 cups mixed baby greens

Servings	1
Prep Time	5 – 6 mins
Cooking Time	10 – 15 mins

PER SERVING

Calories	252
Protein	28 grams
Carbohydrates	22 grams
Fat	5 grams

> Coat the steak with pepper on all sides and press the pepper into the meat. Coat a small skillet in cooking spray and place over medium heat. Add the steak and cook until seared and nicely browned, about 4 minutes, flip and cook for another 5 minutes over medium. Remove from the pan and set aside to cool to room temperature.

> Meanwhile, puncture the sweet potato in a few places with a knife or fork and place in the microwave on high for 5 minutes, turn and heat for another 5 minutes.

> Add the baby greens to a large salad bowl. Once the steak and potatoes have cooled, cut the steak into slices and the potato into chunks. Scatter the mushrooms and potatoes over the greens, then add the steak and top with scallions. Divide into 2 equal portions and top with dressing of your choice.

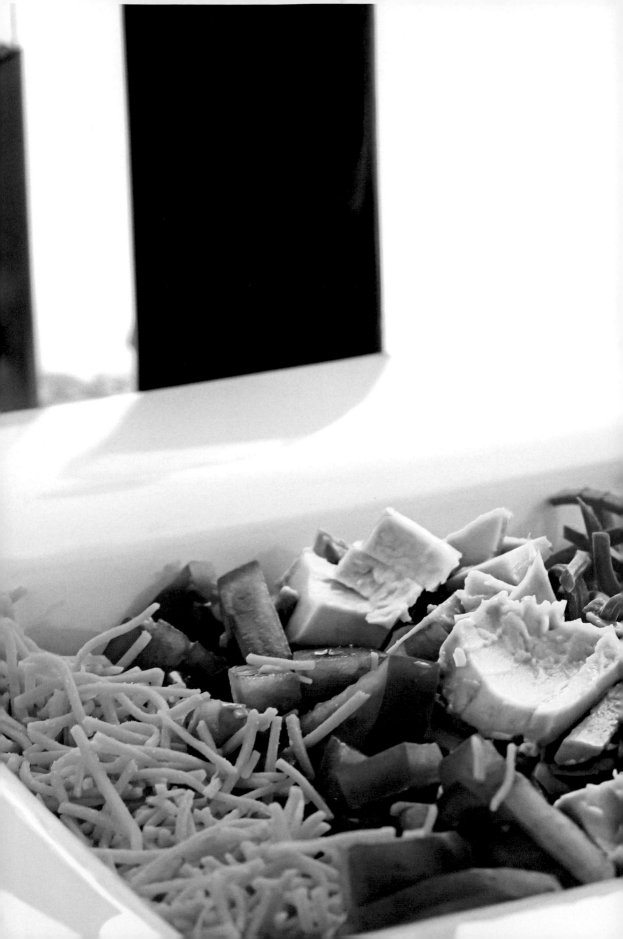

CLASSIC COBB SALAD

Servings	2
Prep Time	5 mins

PER SERVING

Calories	494
Protein	54 grams
Carbohydrates	20 grams
Fat	23 grams

1 small head iceberg lettuce, chopped

2 boneless, skinless chicken breasts (6 ounces each), cooked, and cut into small cubes

2 hardboiled eggs, chopped

2 medium tomatoes, chopped

1 avocado, sliced

1 cup carrots, grated

1/4 cup low-fat mild cheddar cheese, shredded

> Evenly divide the lettuce between two large bowls.

> Toss in the rest of the ingredients and serve with dressing of your choice.

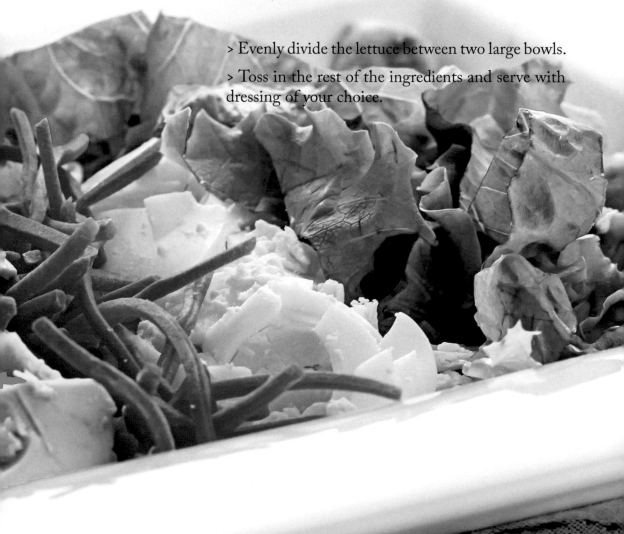

SPINACH & SALMON SALAD

Servings	2
Prep Time	15 mins
Cooking Time	15 – 20 mins

PER SERVING

Calories	395
Protein	42 grams
Carbohydrates	24 grams
Fat	15 grams

2 wild Atlantic salmon fillets (6 ounces each), rinsed and dried

1 teaspoon fresh parsley, chopped, or 1 teaspoon dried parsley

1/2 medium lemon, juiced

1 teaspoon ground black pepper

1 teaspoon extra-virgin olive oil

1 clove garlic, minced

1/2 cup sweet onion, chopped

20 asparagus spears, with bottoms cut off

1/2 yellow bell pepper, cored, seeded, and cut into strips

1 tablespoon honey mustard (use the lowest sodium one you can find)

4 cups spinach leaves

10 grape or cherry tomatoes, halved

1/2 cup blueberries

1 tablespoon slivered almonds

> Choose a skillet that's large enough to allow the salmon to lie flat; you may need to cut the salmon in half to accommodate this.

> Place the salmon in the skillet skin side down, add the parsley, lemon juice, and black pepper. Cover with about 1 inch of water, or enough to come just over the top of the fish.

> Turn the heat on medium and bring the water to a gentle simmer, let simmer for about 10 minutes, or until the fish is opaque. Remove from the heat and cover.

> In a nonstick skillet over medium-high heat, add the oil, garlic, and onion. Cook for about 3 minutes, or until lightly browned. Add the asparagus and bell pepper. Bring the heat down to medium and cook for 2 – 3 minutes longer, or until the veggies are slightly tender. Finish by stirring in the honey mustard and cooking for 30 seconds longer to caramelize.

> Now to prepare the salad, evenly divide your spinach, tomato, and blueberries between two plates. Carefully remove your salmon from the pan and gently scrape off the skin and fat. Top each plate with half of the salmon, lay your veggies on top and sprinkle with almonds.

QUICK & EASY PROTEIN SALAD

Servings	1
Prep Time	15 – 20 mins

PER SERVING

Calories	323
Protein	28 grams
Carbohydrates	29 grams
Fat	13 grams

2 cups baby spring mix

2 scallions, chopped

1/2 cucumber, halved and sliced

4 mushrooms, halved and sliced

1/4 medium avocado, diced

1/2 cup fat-free cottage cheese

1 hardboiled egg, diced

1 lemon, juiced

1 clove garlic, minced

3 tablespoons low-fat buttermilk

salt and ground black pepper, to taste

> Add the spring mix, scallions, cucumber, mushrooms, avocado, cottage cheese, and hardboiled egg to a medium-sized mixing bowl and toss. Transfer to large plate.

> In a small mixing bowl, add the lemon juice, garlic, buttermilk, salt, and pepper and mix well. Pour dressing over salad.

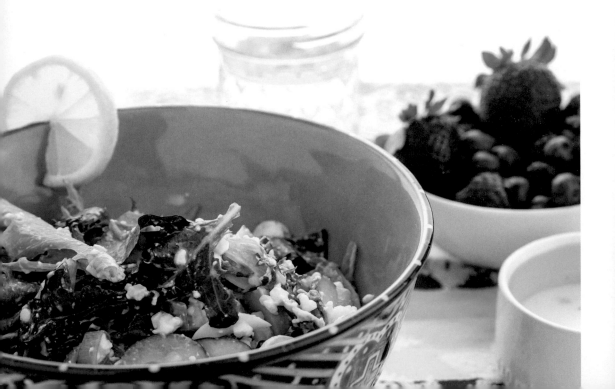

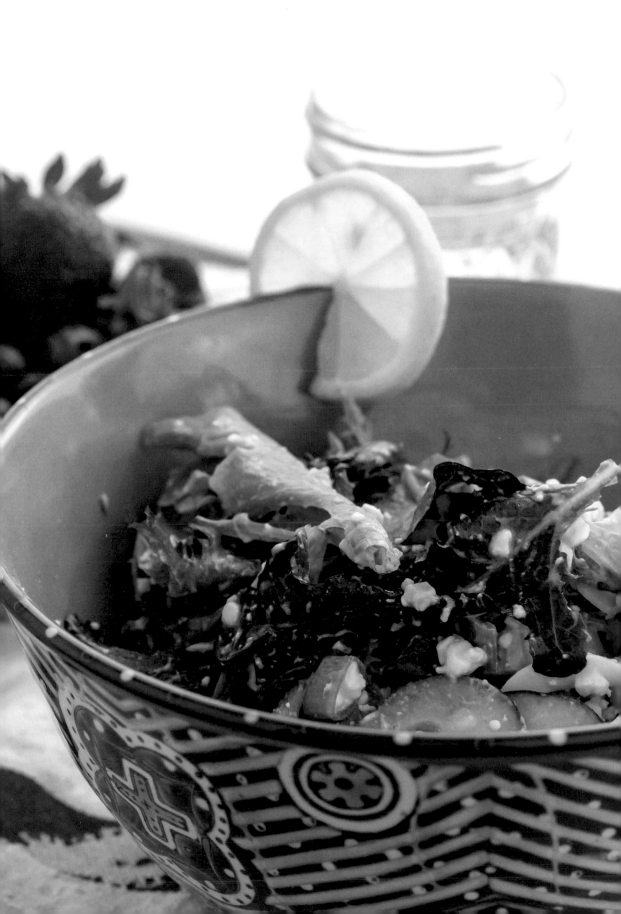

Servings	1
Prep Time	10 mins
PER SERVING	
Calories	351
Protein	42 grams
Carbohydrates	20 grams
Fat	13 grams

TROPICAL CHICKEN SALAD

1 boneless, skinless chicken breast (6 ounces), cooked, and cut into cubes

1/8 cup celery, diced

1/4 cup pineapple, cut into chunks

1/4 cup orange, cut into chunks

1 tablespoon pecans, chopped

1/4 cup seedless grapes, halved

2 cups romaine lettuce

salt and ground black pepper, to taste

> Combine all ingredients except for the lettuce in a large bowl.

> Gently mix until well combined and season with salt and pepper.

> Serve on top of the lettuce leaves.

SIDES

The following side dishes can be included with your meals, not only to add some excitement and variety of taste, but also to help you meet your nutritional requirements. Be creative, mix and match sides with main dishes, and you'll discover food combinations that you'll come back to time and time again.

GREEN BEANS ALMONDINE

Servings	4
Prep Time	Under 5 mins
Cooking Time	5 – 10 mins

PER SERVING

Calories	83
Protein	4 grams
Carbohydrates	10 grams
Fat	5 grams

1 pound fresh green beans, washed and trimmed

1/2 teaspoon extra-virgin olive oil

1/4 cup slivered almonds

salt and ground black pepper, to taste

> Bring a large pot of water to a boil on high heat. Add the green beans and boil for 2 – 4 minutes, or until tender.

> Drain the beans and place in a large bowl. Stir in the oil, salt, and pepper.

> Heat a nonstick skillet over medium-high heat. Coat the almonds in cooking spray and add to hot skillet. Stir frequently for 2 – 3 minutes, or until toasted. Reduce heat to medium and add the green bean mixture. Cook for another 2 minutes, stirring occasionally.

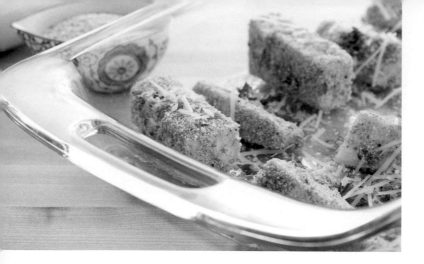

BAKED YELLOW SQUASH

Servings	4
Prep Time	5 mins
Cooking Time	15 – 20 mins

PER SERVING

Calories	75
Protein	6 grams
Carbohydrates	11 grams
Fat	2 grams

1 teaspoon extra-virgin olive oil

2 egg whites

1/2 cup skim milk

2/3 cup low-carb bread crumbs

1 tablespoon Parmesan cheese, shredded

1/2 teaspoon onion powder

1/2 teaspoon paprika

1/2 teaspoon dried parsley

1/2 teaspoon garlic powder

1/4 teaspoon ground black pepper

2 large yellow squash, quarter-cut lengthwise, then cut in half widthwise

> Preheat the oven to 450°F.

> In medium-sized bowl, lightly whisk the egg whites and milk.

> In a different medium-sized bowl, add the bread crumbs, cheese, onion powder, paprika, parsley, garlic powder, and pepper. Mix well.

> Dunk the squash in the egg mixture and then coat in the bread crumb mixture.

> Coat a baking dish in the oil and add the eggplant cut side up. Place in the oven for 15 minutes, or until browned.

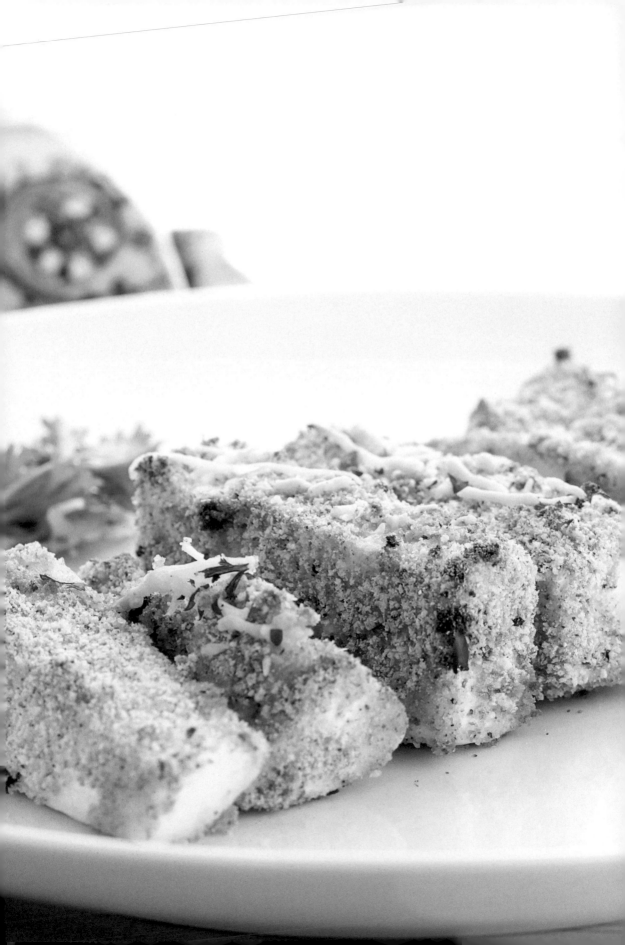

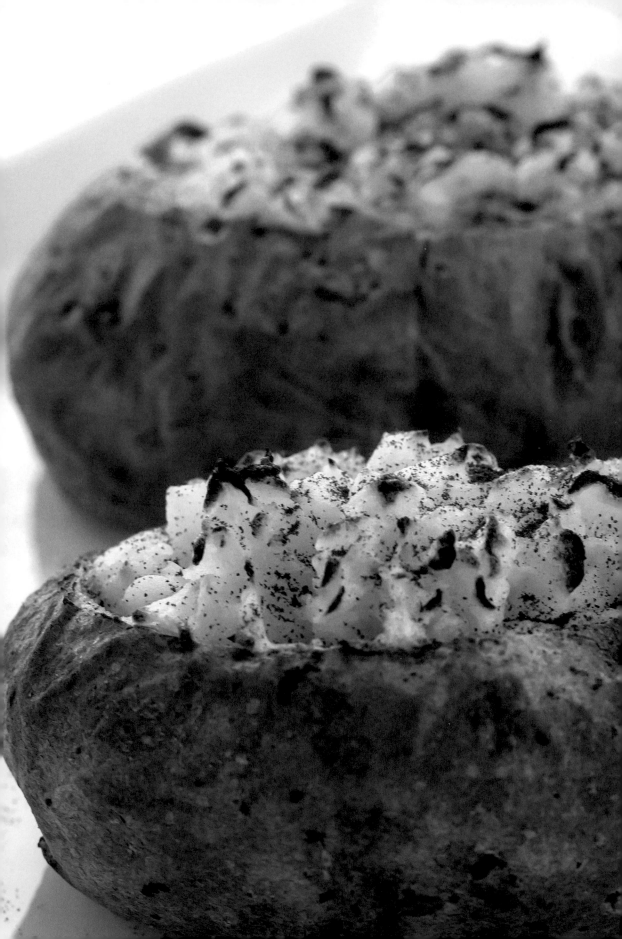

ROASTED GARLIC TWICE-BAKED POTATO

Servings	6
Prep Time	5 mins
Cooking Time	1 hr 20 – 30 mins

PER SERVING

Calories	216
Protein	6 grams
Carbohydrates	39 grams
Fat	5 grams

6 medium-sized baking potatoes

1 whole garlic bulb

1 teaspoon extra-virgin olive oil

2 tablespoons unsalted butter, softened

1/2 cup skim milk

1/2 cup low-fat buttermilk

1 1/2 teaspoons fresh rosemary, minced

1/2 teaspoon salt

1/2 teaspoon ground black pepper

dash of paprika

> Place the potatoes on a baking sheet and bake at 400°F for 45 – 55 minutes, or until tender.

> Meanwhile, remove the outer papery skin from garlic, drizzle with oil and wrap in 2 sheets of heavy-duty foil. Add the garlic to the oven for 30 – 35 minutes or until softened. Let garlic and potatoes cool for about 10 minutes.

> Once cool enough to handle, cut a thin slice off the top of each potato and discard. Scoop out the pulp until just a thin shell remains, place the pulp in a large mixing bowl, add the softened butter and mash.

> Cut the top off of the garlic head, leaving the root intact, and squeeze the softened garlic into the bowl with the potatoes, add the milk, buttermilk, rosemary, salt, and pepper and mix well.

> Spoon the potato mixture back into the shells and place back on the baking sheet. Bake at 425°F for 20 – 25 minutes, or until heated through. Remove from oven and add a dash of paprika to each top.

SWEET POTATO CHIPS

2 medium-sized sweet potatoes, peeled and thinly sliced

1 tablespoon extra-virgin olive oil

1/2 teaspoon salt

Servings	6
Prep Time	5 mins
Cooking Time	25 mins, or until crispy

PER SERVING

Calories	82
Protein	1 gram
Carbohydrates	12 grams
Fat	4 grams

> Position one rack in the center and one in the lower position of the oven and preheat oven to 400°F.

> Place the sweet potatoes in a large bowl and drizzle olive oil over top, toss to coat well. Spread potatoes evenly over 2 baking sheets and place in oven. Bake, flipping once half way through, until centers are soft and edges are slightly crispy, about 22 – 25 minutes. Sprinkle salt over top.

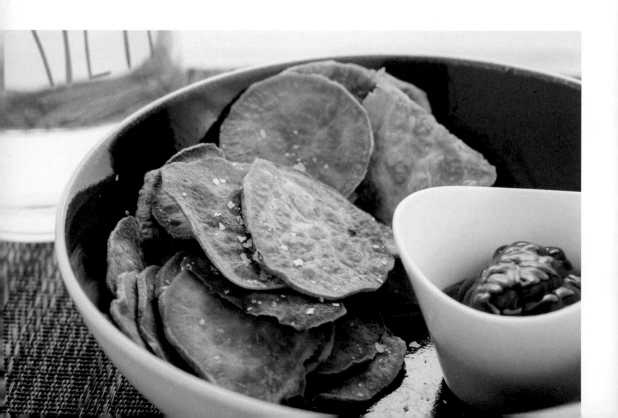

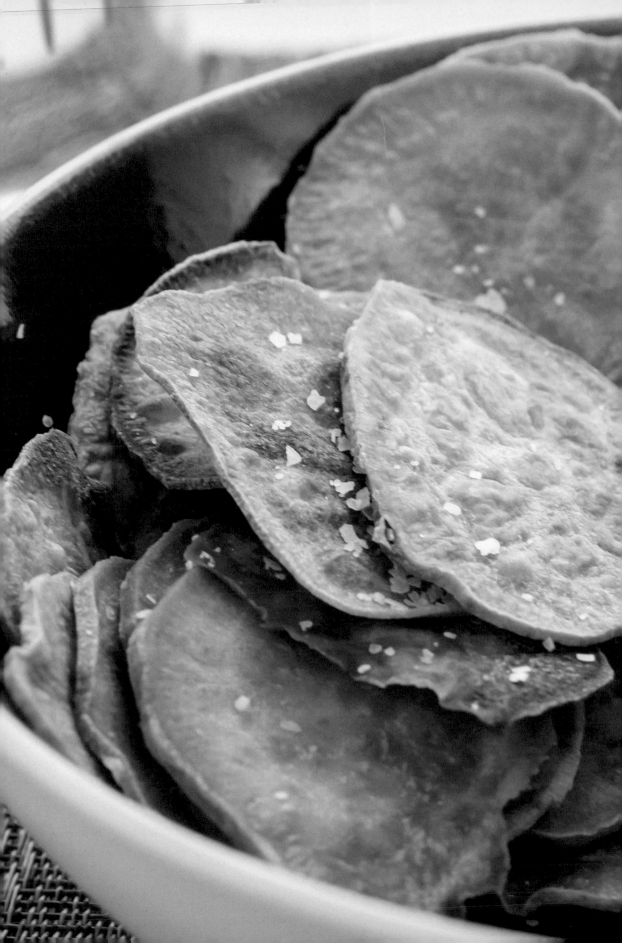

MIKE'S DELICIOUS BROWN RICE

Servings	4
Prep Time	Under 5 mins
Cooking Time	50 mins – 1 hr

PER SERVING

Calories	291
Protein	8 grams
Carbohydrates	42 grams
Fat	10 grams

1 cup long-grain brown rice

2 cups low-sodium chicken broth

1/2 cup carrots, shredded

1/2 cup zucchini, shredded

3 tablespoons sunflower kernels

3 tablespoons sliced almonds

1/4 teaspoon red pepper flakes

2 tablespoons fresh parsley, minced

> Add the rice to the chicken broth and bring to a boil. Reduce heat to medium-low and cover with a tight fitting lid, let cook for 50 minutes.

> Remove rice from heat and let sit covered for 10 minutes.

> When the rice is almost finished, coat a large skillet in cooking spray and place over medium-high heat. Add the carrot and zucchini and sauté for 2 minutes. Add the sunflower kernels, almonds, and red pepper flakes and cook until the almonds are browned.

> Add the rice and parsley, combine ingredients well, and sauté for 1 minute so flavors can mix.

MUSHROOM RISOTTO

Servings	4
Prep Time	Under 5 mins
Cooking Time	15 – 20 mins

PER SERVING

Calories	255
Protein	12 grams
Carbohydrates	49 grams
Fat	3 grams

1 cup Arborio rice

3 small onions, finely chopped

1 clove garlic, crushed

1 teaspoon fresh parsley, minced

salt and ground black pepper, to taste

1 1/2 cups fresh mushrooms, sliced

1 cup skim milk

1/4 cup fat-free half and half

3 cups low-sodium chicken broth

1 teaspoon unsalted butter

1/2 cup low-fat Parmesan cheese, grated

> Coat a large skillet in cooking spray and place over medium-high heat. Add the onion and garlic and sauté until onion is tender. Remove the crushed garlic and stir in the parsley, salt, pepper, and mushrooms. Reduce heat to low and cook until mushrooms have softened.

> Add the milk and cream to the skillet, mix everything, then stir in the rice. Bring to a simmer, then stir in the chicken broth one cup at a time, until it is absorbed by the rice.

> Once the rice is finished cooking, stir in the butter and cheese, let cheese melt for a minute, then remove from heat.

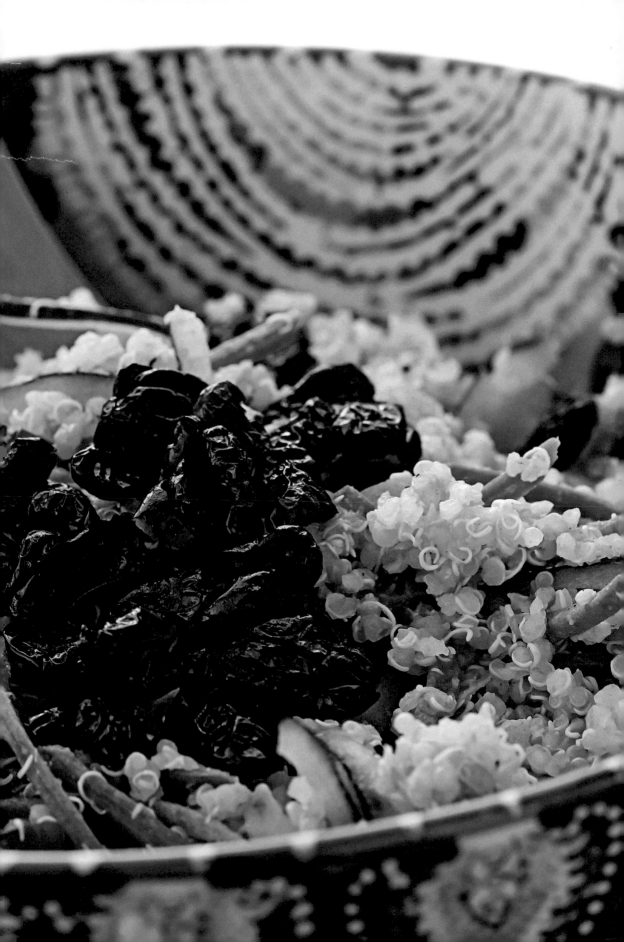

CRANBERRY QUINOA SALAD

Servings	4
Prep Time	5 mins
Cooking Time	15 – 20 mins
PER SERVING	
Calories	287
Protein	8 grams
Carbohydrates	51 grams
Fat	7 grams

1 cup quinoa, rinsed

1 1/2 cups water

1/4 cup red bell pepper, chopped

1/4 cup yellow bell pepper, chopped

1 small red onion, finely chopped

1 1/2 teaspoons curry powder

1/4 cup fresh cilantro, chopped

1 lime, juiced

1/4 cup sliced almonds, toasted

1/2 cup carrots, minced

1/2 cup dried cranberries

salt and ground black pepper, to taste

> Pour the water in a large saucepan, cover with a tight fitting lid, and place over high heat. Once water starts to boil, pour in the quinoa, reduce heat to low, and cover. Simmer until the water has been absorbed, about 15 – 20 minutes. Transfer the quinoa to a large mixing bowl and place in the refrigerator until cold.

> Once the quinoa is chilled, stir in the bell peppers, red onion, curry powder, cilantro, lime juice, sliced almonds, carrots, cranberries, salt, and pepper.

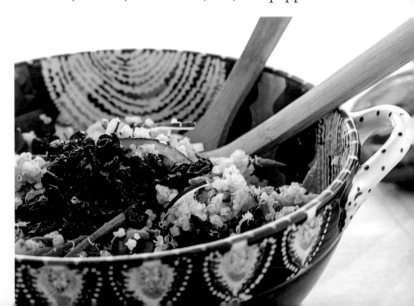

COUSCOUS SALAD

Servings	8
Prep Time	5 – 10 mins
Cooking Time	5 mins

PER SERVING

Calories	222
Protein	8 grams
Carbohydrates	40 grams
Fat	3 grams

1 box (12 ounces) couscous

8 leaves Bibb lettuce

2 lemons, juiced

1/2 teaspoon lemon zest

2 tablespoons honey

1 tablespoon Dijon mustard

1 teaspoon extra-virgin olive oil

1 container (3.5 ounces) low-fat feta cheese, crumbled

3 plum tomatoes, chopped

1 medium cucumber, peeled and cut into chunks

1/2 onion, finely chopped

1 can (2.25 ounces) sliced black olives, drained and rinsed

1/4 teaspoon ground black pepper

1/2 cup fresh parsley, chopped

> Bring a pot of lightly salted water to a boil. Place your couscous in a separate bowl; add the boiling water and mix well. Cover and cook for about 5 minutes, or according to package instructions.

> Meanwhile, place the lettuce leaves on 8 separate plates.

> In a small bowl, add your lemon juice, lemon zest, honey, mustard, and oil. Whisk to combine the ingredients well.

> In a different bowl, combine the cooked couscous, cheese, tomatoes, cucumber, onion, olives, pepper, and parsley. Once mixed, stir in the lemon juice mixture.

> Top the lettuce with equal amounts of the couscous salad. This dish can be served warm or refrigerated and served chilled.

Servings	6
Prep Time	Under 5 mins
Cooking Time	5 – 7 mins
PER SERVING	
Calories	109
Protein	4 grams
Carbohydrates	20 grams
Fat	2 grams

LEMON AND CILANTRO QUINOA

1 cup quinoa, rinsed

1/4 cup fresh lemon juice

1/2 cup fresh cilantro, chopped

> Prepare the quinoa according to package directions. Once cooked, add the lemon juice and fresh cilantro. Mix well and serve.

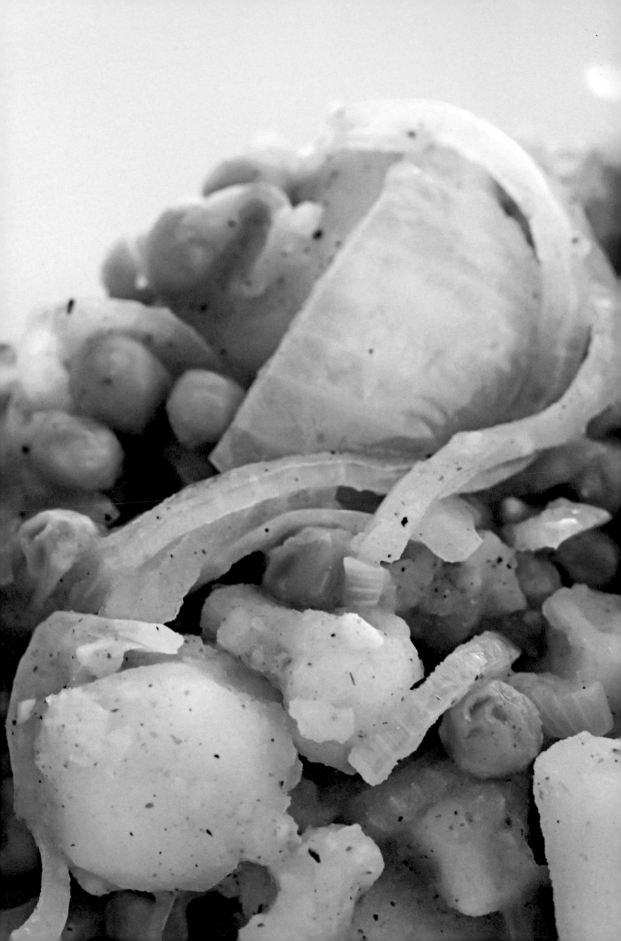

CURRY POTATOES AND CAULIFLOWER

Servings	4
Prep Time	Under 5 mins
Cooking Time	25 mins

PER SERVING

Calories	234
Protein	10 grams
Carbohydrates	50 grams
Fat	1 gram

1 cauliflower head (2 – 3 pounds), cut into florets

1 pound (around 3 medium) potatoes, peeled and cut into 1-inch cubes

1 medium onion, chopped

2 cloves garlic, crushed

2 tablespoons garam masala or curry powder

1 cup low-sodium vegetable broth

2 cups frozen peas

> Bring a pot of lightly salted water to a boil. Add the cauliflower and potatoes and cook for 4 – 5 minutes. Drain.

> Meanwhile, coat a Dutch oven in cooking spray and place over medium heat. Add chopped onion and garlic and cook 2 – 3 minutes, or until the onions are softened. Add the garam masala and stir for 1 minute.

> Add the cooked potatoes and cauliflower and stir well, coating in the onion mixture, add the vegetable broth and use it to deglaze (scrape the bottom of the Dutch oven and remove any stuck bits). Cover and let simmer for 10 minutes. Add the peas, mix well, and cover for another 5 – 7 minutes.

VEGETABLE SAUTÉ

1 tablespoon extra-virgin olive oil

2 cloves garlic, crushed

2 medium zucchini, cut in half, then into sticks

2 cups grape tomatoes

3 cups baby spinach

1 tablespoon fresh lemon juice

pinch of ground black pepper

Servings	6
Prep Time	5 mins
Cooking Time	10 mins
PER SERVING	
Calories	46
Protein	2 grams
Carbohydrates	5 grams
Fat	3 grams

> Heat the oil in a pan on medium-low heat. Add the garlic and cook for 1 minute, stir in the zucchini and raise the heat to medium.

> Cook for 3 – 4 minutes, stir in the tomatoes, cook for another minute, then stir in the spinach. Cook for another 3 – 4 minutes, then stir in the lemon juice and black pepper.

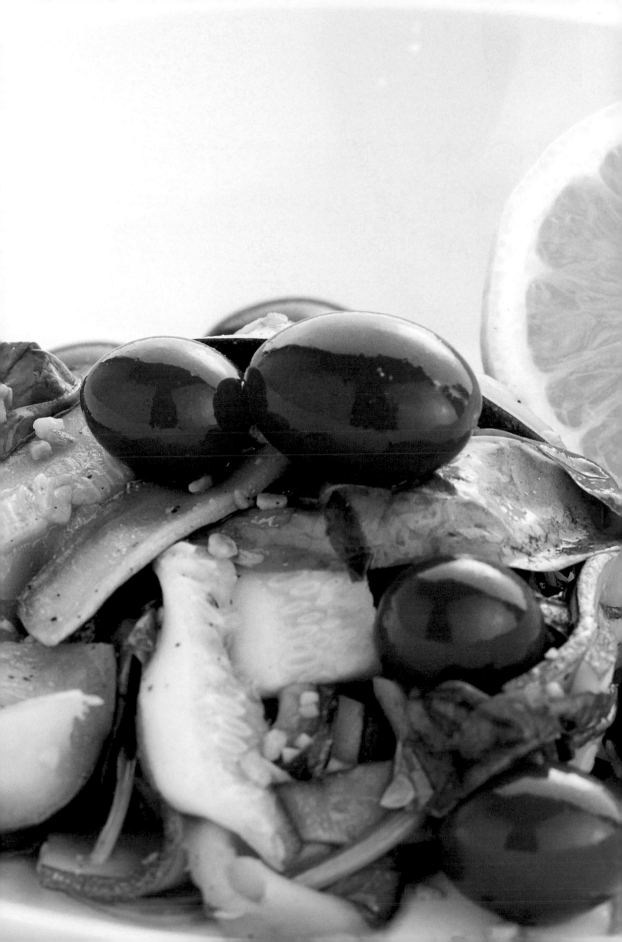

BROWN RICE PILAF

Servings	4
Prep Time	5 – 10 mins
Cooking Time	40 – 45 mins

PER SERVING

Calories	210
Protein	5 grams
Carbohydrates	38 grams
Fat	4 grams

1 tablespoon unsalted butter

1 shallot, chopped

1 cup long-grain brown rice, rinsed

salt and ground black pepper, to taste

2 cups low-sodium chicken broth

1 clove garlic, smashed

2 sprigs fresh thyme

3 tablespoons fresh flat-leaf parsley, chopped

3 scallions, thinly sliced

> Melt the butter in a large pan over medium heat. Add the shallot and cook for 1 – 2 minutes, until tender. Add the rice and stir well, coating with the butter and shallot mixture. Cook for a few minutes, until the rice is glossy. Add salt and pepper.

> Stir in the chicken broth, garlic, and thyme. Cover with a tight fitting lid and cook for 40 minutes. Remove from the heat and let sit for 10 minutes. Remove the thyme sprigs and garlic clove (optional). Fluff the rice with a spoon or fork and stir in the parsley and scallions.

HEALTHY SWEET POTATO CASSEROLE

Servings	6
Prep Time	10 – 15 mins
Cooking Time	30 mins
PER SERVING	
Calories	292
Protein	7 grams
Carbohydrates	56 grams
Fat	5 grams

3 cups sweet potatoes, cooked and mashed

1/3 cup packed brown sugar

1/3 cup skim milk

2 tablespoons butter, melted

1 teaspoon vanilla extract

1/2 teaspoon salt

2 egg whites

1/2 cup packed brown sugar

1/4 cup all-purpose flour

2 tablespoons butter, chilled

> Preheat the oven to 350°F.

> Coat a 2-quart baking dish with cooking spray.

> In a large mixing bowl, add the mashed sweet potatoes, 1/3 cup brown sugar, skim milk, melted butter, vanilla extract, salt, and egg whites. Mix well and transfer to the baking dish, spreading evenly.

> In a medium-sized mixing bowl, add the 1/2 cup brown sugar and flour. Slowly add in the 2 tablespoons chilled butter and stir until the mixture has the consistency of coarse crumbs.

> Sprinkle the crumb mixture over the sweet potatoes and bake for 30 minutes.

SQUASH &
BROCCOLI
STIR-FRY

Servings	6
Prep Time	10 mins
Cooking Time	10 – 15 mins

PER SERVING

Calories	82
Protein	2 grams
Carbohydrates	15 grams
Fat	3 grams

1 pound butternut squash, peeled, seeded and cut into 1/4-inch slices

1 garlic clove, minced

1/4 teaspoon ground ginger

1 cup broccoli florets

1/2 cup celery, thinly sliced

1/2 cup onion, thinly sliced

2 teaspoons honey

1 tablespoon lemon juice

2 tablespoons sunflower kernels

> Coat a large skillet with cooking spray and place over medium-high heat. Add the squash, garlic, and ginger and stir-fry for 3 minutes. Add the broccoli, celery, and onion, and continue to stir-fry for 3 – 4 minutes or until all the vegetables are tender.

> Meanwhile, in a small bowl, combine the honey and lemon juice and mix well.

> Place the vegetables in a large serving dish and pour the honey mixture over, toss to coat. Sprinkle the sunflower kernels on top.

PROTEIN SHAKES

Protein shakes are a great way to help meet daily nutritional requirements, and are especially good for your post-workout meal due to fast absorption of the protein and high-glycemic carbs.

I recommend that you use a high-quality whey (I like Optimum Nutrition's Natural Whey) or egg (I like Healthy 'n Fit's 100% Egg Protein) protein powder because both taste pretty good and have no artificial sweeteners. Casein is also a good option for your before-bed protein due to its slow absorption rate (this helps you make it through the night with minimal catabolism).

I don't recommend weight-gainer proteins unless you need to occasionally slam down a post-workout meal fast and don't even have time to make a proper shake.

If you're going to be making several shakes per day (and most of us do), I recommend that you simply mix the powder with water and then get your carbs from fruit or other sources. The shake recipes given in this section require a blender and other ingredients, and are more suited for your post-workout meals (most of these contain 50+ grams of carbs), or as a meal replacement.

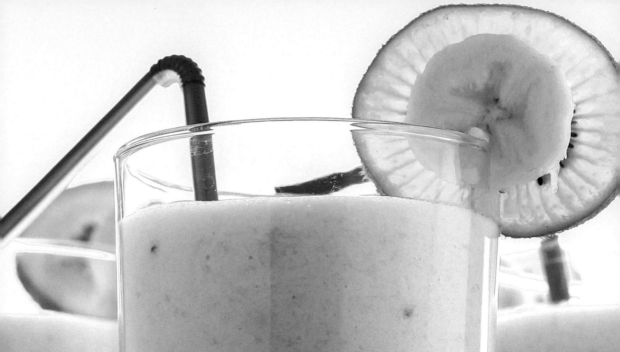

KIWI-BANANA-
MANGO MONSTER
SHAKE

1/2 medium kiwi, peeled and sliced

1/2 medium banana, sliced

1/2 medium mango, peeled and diced

1/2 cup fresh or canned pineapple, diced

1 scoop vanilla whey protein powder

1 cup skim milk

1/2 cup papaya, diced

1 lemon, juiced

1/2 tablespoon clover honey

1 packet (1 gram) stevia or other sugar alternative

Servings	1
Prep Time	15 mins
PER SERVING	
Calories	459
Protein	35 grams
Carbohydrates	78 grams
Fat	2 grams

> Place all of your ingredients in a blender, blend on high until desired consistency.

CHOCOLATE ALMOND MOCHA SHAKE

Servings	1
Prep Time	Under 5 mins

PER SERVING

Calories	397
Protein	55 grams
Carbohydrates	16 grams
Fat	13 grams

1/2 cup skim milk

1 tablespoon instant coffee

10 unsalted almonds

1 tablespoon lecithin granules

2 packets (2 grams) stevia or other sugar alternative

2 scoops chocolate whey protein powder

1 cup crushed ice or 6 – 8 ice cubes

> Start blending all of your ingredients except the ice on high. Once mixed, turn the blender to medium and add your ice cubes until desired consistency.

POST-WORKOUT PEANUT BUTTER BLAST

Servings	1
Prep Time	5 mins

PER SERVING

Calories	810
Protein	68 grams
Carbohydrates	70 grams
Fat	27 grams

1 1/2 cups skim milk

1 tablespoon vanilla extract

1 tablespoon flaxseed oil

1 teaspoon L-glutamine powder

1 tablespoon micronized creatine monohydrate

1 tablespoon peanut butter

1/4 cup old-fashioned oats

1 cup crushed ice or 6 – 8 ice cubes

2 scoops vanilla or chocolate whey protein powder

1 banana, frozen

> Start blending all of your ingredients except the banana and protein powder on high. Once mixed, turn the blender to medium and add your banana and protein powder, blend until desired consistency.

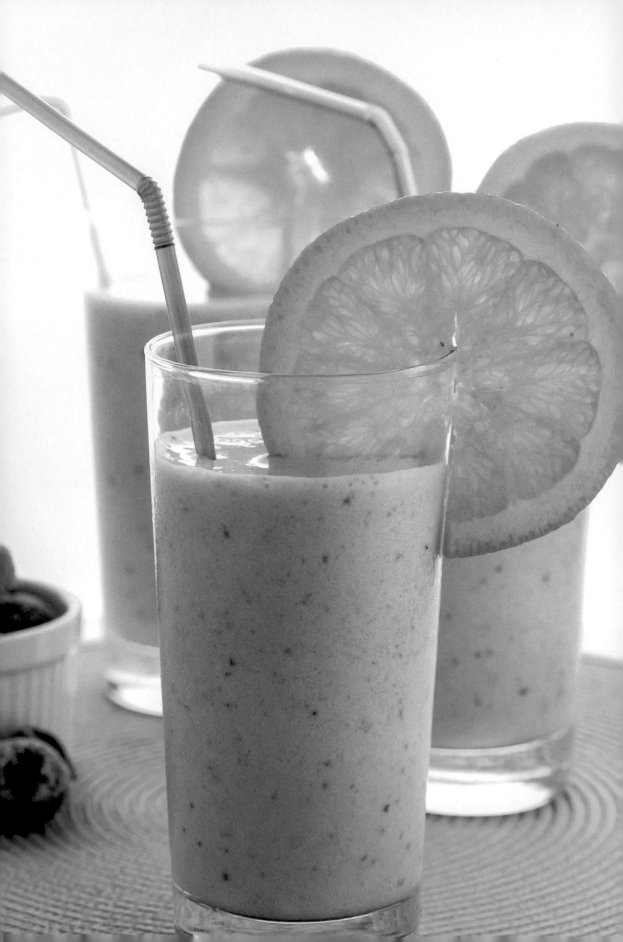

ORANGE JULIUS

Servings	1
Prep Time	5 mins
PER SERVING	
Calories	453
Protein	51 grams
Carbohydrates	50 grams
Fat	3 grams

2 scoops vanilla whey protein powder

1 cup orange juice

3/4 cup crushed ice or 4 – 6 ice cubes

1 tablespoon vanilla extract

1/2 medium banana

3 strawberries, frozen

2 packets (2 grams) of stevia or other sugar alternative

> Place all ingredients in blender and blend on medium speed until desired consistency.

PROTEIN BARS & SNACKS

Meeting your daily caloric and nutritional requirements is going to mean eating "snack" meals in between your breakfasts, lunches, and dinners. You might have to change your definition of "snack," however.

When I say "snack," I don't mean crackers, cookies, muffins, cereal, doughnuts, chips, pretzels, ice cream, candy, or any other tempting little late-night nibbles. If you have any of these nutritionally bankrupt foods in your home, I recommend you throw them out right now. Yes, all of them, because at best they're "empty" calories and at worst, actually harmful to your muscle-building or fat-loss ambitions.

Instead, you should stock up on healthy snacks such as low-fat cottage cheese, fresh fruits and vegetables, low-fat or fat-free yogurt, nuts, and granola.

What about protein bars for snacks? Most protein bars sold in stores are better snacks than Snickers bars, but that's not saying much.

The problem with most protein bars is they contain a large amount of junk carbs such as sugar and high fructose corn syrup, and not much protein (and to make matters even worse, some companies selling these bars claim they have more protein than they do!). Most bars also contain artificial sweeteners such as sucralose or aspartame, chemicals to enhance the taste, and chemical preservatives. There's just too much junk in most to make them worth eating.

In this section of the book, I'm going to show you how to make your own delicious protein bars using healthy, high-quality ingredients, along with a few other yummy snacks.

CHOCOLATE PEANUT BUTTER PROTEIN BARS

Servings	8 (1 bar per serving)
Prep Time	5 mins

PER SERVING

Calories	278
Protein	20 grams
Carbohydrates	27 grams
Fat	11 grams

3 cups old-fashioned oats

1/2 cup peanut butter

1 cup skim milk

4 scoops chocolate or vanilla whey protein powder

dash of cinnamon

1 tablespoon stevia or other sugar alternative

> Combine all of the ingredients except the stevia in a large bowl and mix until a sticky batter is formed. Coat a shallow baking dish in cooking spray and spread the mixture out over the dish.

> Evenly sprinkle the stevia over the mixture and place in the fridge overnight. Cut into 8 equal bars.

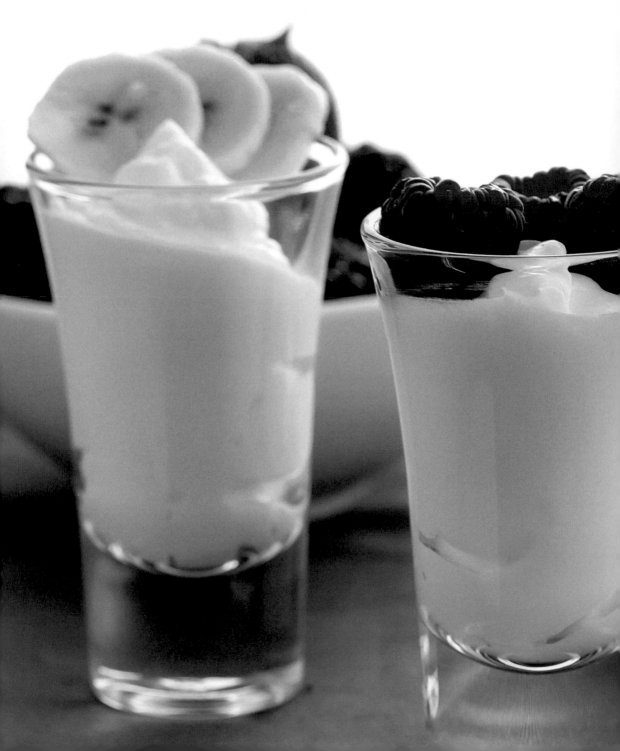

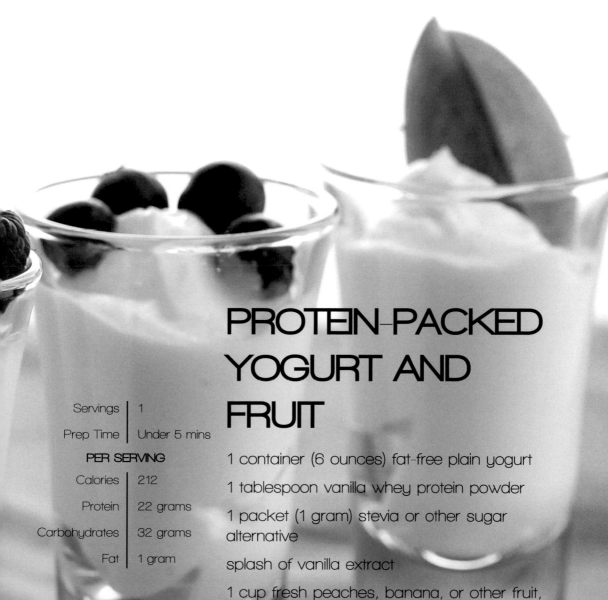

PROTEIN-PACKED YOGURT AND FRUIT

Servings	1
Prep Time	Under 5 mins

PER SERVING

Calories	212
Protein	22 grams
Carbohydrates	32 grams
Fat	1 gram

1 container (6 ounces) fat-free plain yogurt

1 tablespoon vanilla whey protein powder

1 packet (1 gram) stevia or other sugar alternative

splash of vanilla extract

1 cup fresh peaches, banana, or other fruit, chopped

> Mix the yogurt, protein powder, stevia, and vanilla extract in a medium bowl. Stir until fully combined.

> Top with fruit.

PROTEIN PUDDING BARS

8 scoops chocolate or vanilla whey protein powder

3 cups old-fashioned oats

1 package sugar-free fat-free pudding (use same flavor as protein)

2 cups skim milk

Servings	8 (1 bar per serving)
Prep Time	5 mins
PER SERVING	
Calories	284
Protein	31 grams
Carbohydrates	30 grams
Fat	4 grams

> Combine all ingredients in a large bowl and mix until a sticky batter is formed. Coat a shallow baking dish in cooking spray and spread the mixture out over the dish.

> Place in the refrigerator overnight, cut into 8 equal bars once set.

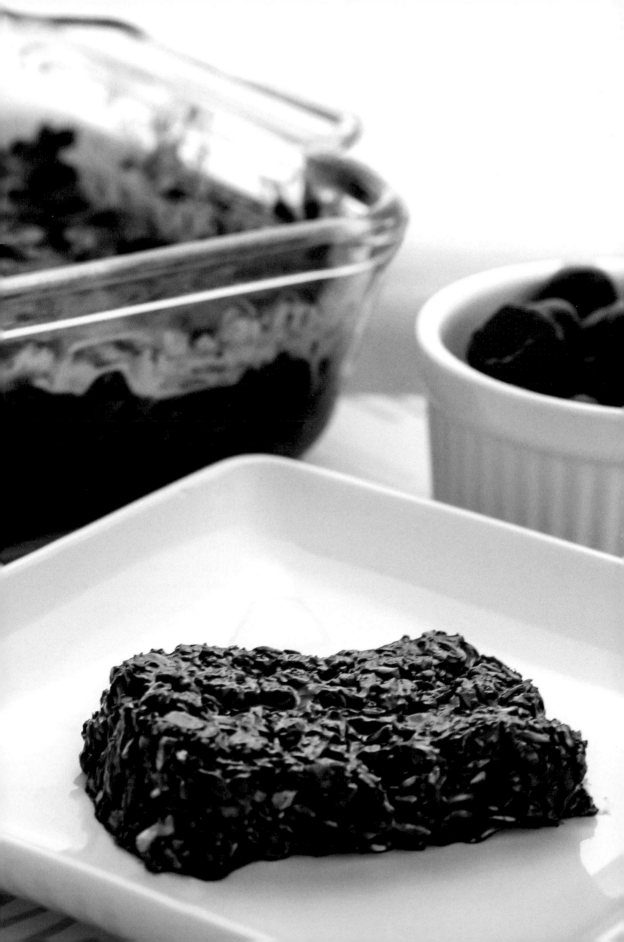

STRAWBERRY BANANA PROTEIN BARS

Servings	8 (1 bar per serving)
Prep Time	5 – 10 mins
Cooking Time	35 – 40 mins

PER SERVING

Calories	199
Protein	22 grams
Carbohydrates	16 grams
Fat	5 grams

1 cup old-fashioned oats

6 scoops strawberry whey protein powder

1/2 cup fat-free dry milk powder

1/4 cup fat-free cream cheese

2 egg whites

1 1/2 bananas, mashed

1/4 cup water

2 tablespoons canola oil

> Preheat the oven to 325°F.

> Spray a shallow baking dish with cooking spray. In a medium-sized mixing bowl, add the oatmeal, protein powder, and dry milk. In a separate medium-sized mixing bowl, combine the cream cheese, egg whites, bananas, water, and oil and beat with an electric hand mixer until thoroughly combined. Slowly add in the dry mixture and beat until fully combined.

> Pour the batter into the prepared baking dish and bake for 30 – 35 minutes, or until a toothpick inserted into the middle comes out clean.

NO-FAT TZATZIKI SAUCE

1/2 large cucumber

3/4 cup plain fat-free yogurt

1/4 tablespoon Worcestershire sauce

1/8 cup fresh mint, finely chopped

salt, to taste

Servings	16 (2 tablespoons per serving)
Prep Time	Under 5 mins

PER SERVING

Calories	12
Protein	1 gram
Carbohydrates	2 grams
Fat	0 grams

> Peel the cucumber and cut in half lengthwise, scoop out the seeds. Finely slice half the cucumber and place into a large mixing bowl. Take the other half and puree in a food processor or blender, add to the mixing bowl.

> Add the remaining ingredients to the mixing bowl and mix well. For guaranteed freshness I recommend using within 3 days.

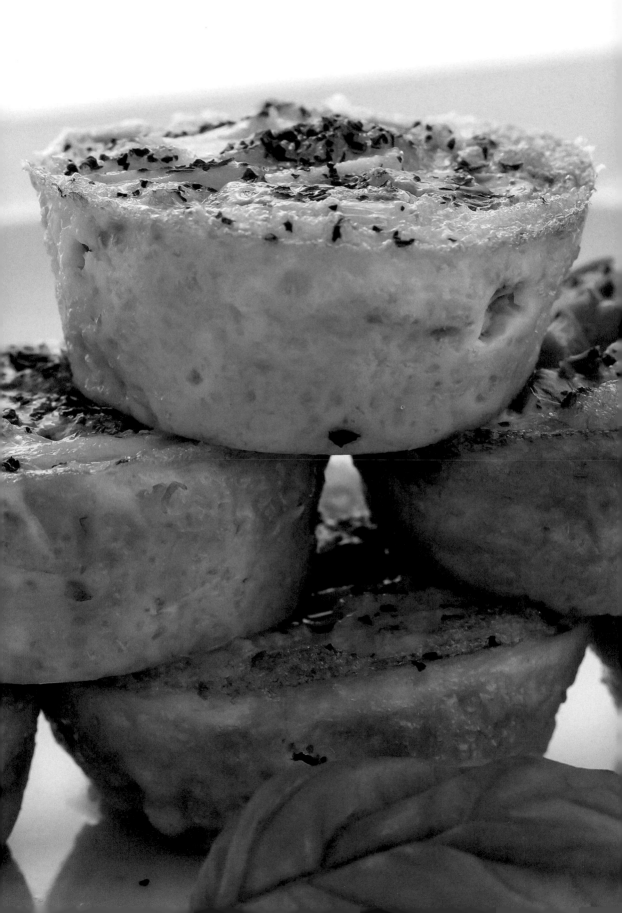

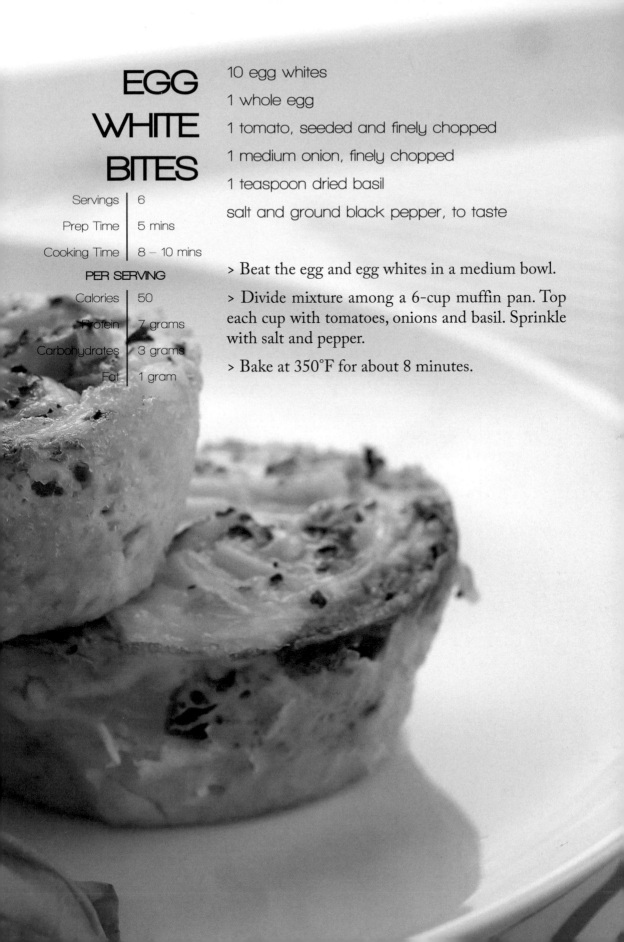

EGG WHITE BITES

Servings	6
Prep Time	5 mins
Cooking Time	8 – 10 mins

PER SERVING

Calories	50
Protein	7 grams
Carbohydrates	3 grams
Fat	1 gram

10 egg whites

1 whole egg

1 tomato, seeded and finely chopped

1 medium onion, finely chopped

1 teaspoon dried basil

salt and ground black pepper, to taste

> Beat the egg and egg whites in a medium bowl.

> Divide mixture among a 6-cup muffin pan. Top each cup with tomatoes, onions and basil. Sprinkle with salt and pepper.

> Bake at 350°F for about 8 minutes.

MEAN GREEN SALSA

Servings	4 (1 cup per serving)
Prep Time	5 – 10 mins

PER SERVING

Calories	141
Protein	4 grams
Carbohydrates	17 grams
Fat	8 grams

2 poblano chili peppers, halved and seeded

2 serrano chili peppers, halved and seeded

1 avocado

1 clove garlic

1 cup cilantro, chopped

1/2 green bell pepper, seeded and chopped

1/2 medium sweet onion, chopped

1/4 head iceberg lettuce, chopped

1/2 cup water

2 limes, juiced

1 can (14.5 ounces) no-salt diced tomatoes, drained

> Place all of your ingredients excluding the tomatoes in a blender or food processor. Blend until mostly smooth with some chunks. If you can't fit it all at once you can blend in multiple batches.

> Pour into a large bowl and add the tomatoes, mix well.

SIZZLING SALSA

Servings	8 (1 cup per serving)
Prep Time	5 – 10 mins

PER SERVING

Calories	58
Protein	1 gram
Carbohydrates	10 grams
Fat	2 grams

6 medium vine-ripened tomatoes, chopped

4 sticks of celery, chopped

4 jalapeño peppers, finely diced

4 serrano or other chili peppers, finely diced (optional)

1 bunch cilantro, finely chopped

1/2 yellow bell pepper, seeded and chopped

1 cup mango, chopped (optional)

1/2 cup sweet onion, chopped

1/2 cup key lime juice

1 tablespoon extra-virgin olive oil

pinch of ground black pepper

> Place all of your ingredients in a large bowl, toss, and serve.

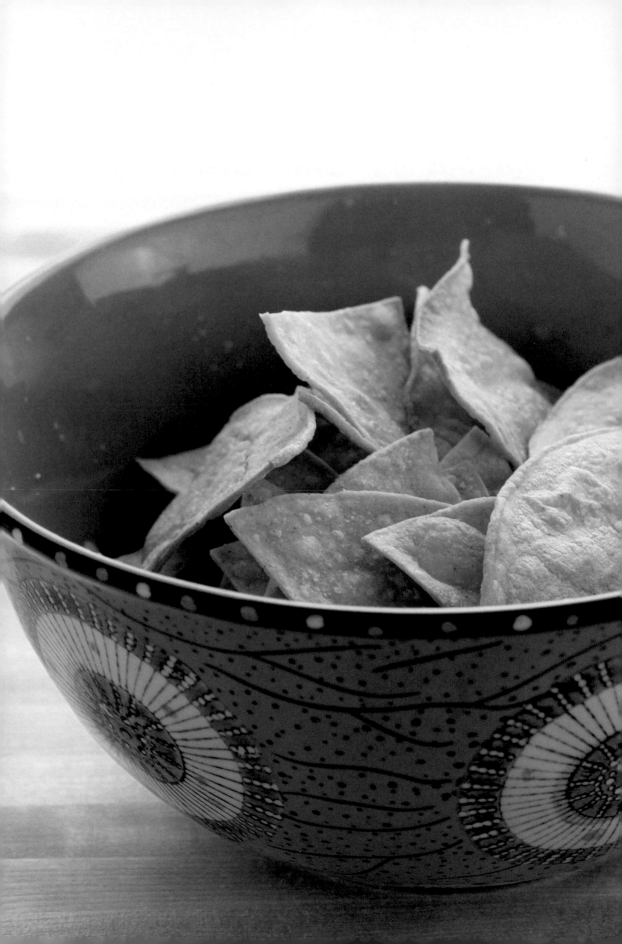

CORN TORTILLA CHIPS

Servings	1
Prep Time	Under 5 mins
Cooking Time	10 mins
PER SERVING	
Calories	80
Protein	2 grams
Carbohydrates	16 grams
Fat	2 grams

Cooking spray

2 (6-inch) corn tortillas

> Preheat the oven to 350°F.

> Cut the tortillas into 6 wedges and place the pieces on a baking sheet. Lightly spray both sides of the chips with cooking spray and bake for 10 minutes, or until crispy and browned on edges.

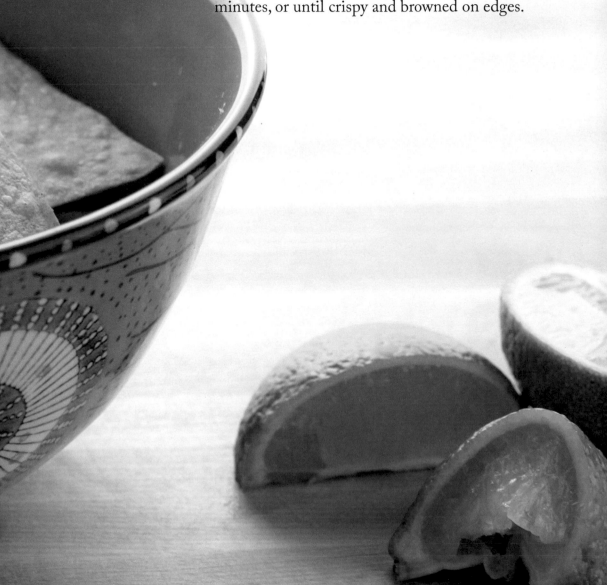

PERFECT GUACAMOLE

Servings	2
Prep Time	5 – 10 mins
PER SERVING	
Calories	295
Protein	6 grams
Carbohydrates	19 grams
Fat	26 grams

2 ripe avocados

1/2 red onion, finely chopped

2 serrano chilies, seeded and finely chopped

1/4 cup fresh cilantro, chopped

1 tablespoon fresh lime juice

1/2 teaspoon salt

dash of ground black pepper

> Cut the avocados in half, pit them and scoop out the peel and place in a mixing bowl. Add in the chopped onion, cilantro, lime, salt, pepper, and half the chili.

> Mash together, I personally like mine slightly chunky, so I don't mash too much. Taste, add additional lime, salt, and chili to reach desired flavor and level of spice. I always end up adding a tiny bit more salt and the rest of the chili, but that's just how I like it!

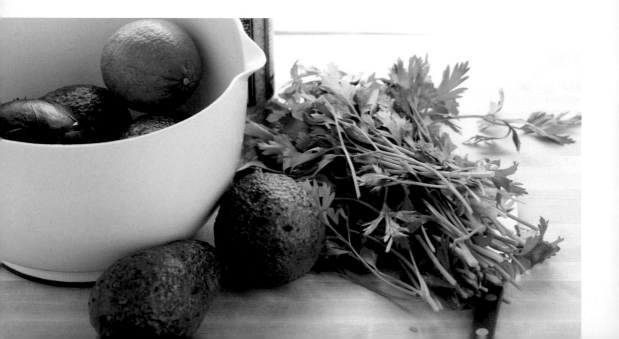

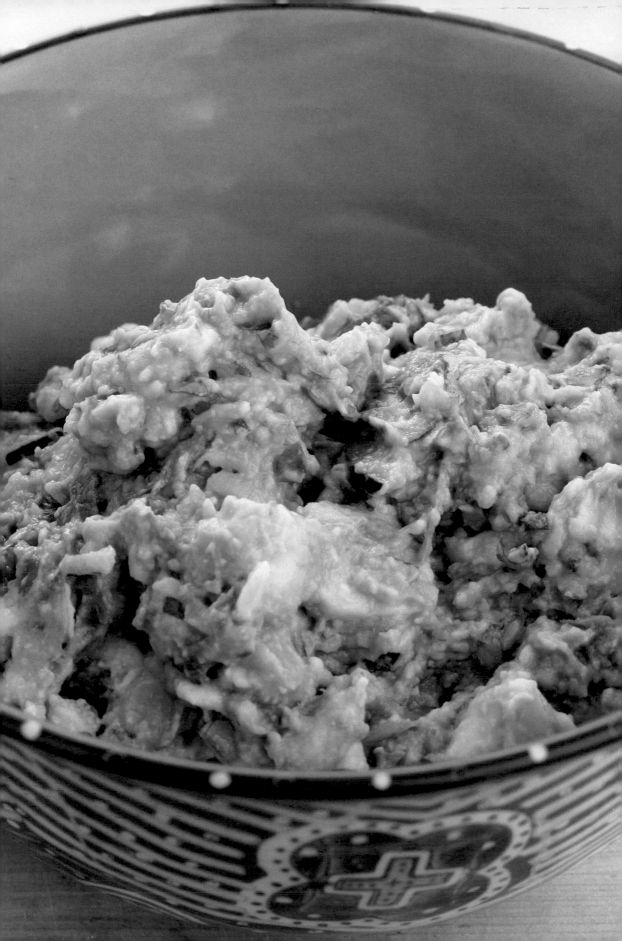

GARLIC VEGETABLE DIP

1 cup fat-free sour cream

2 tablespoons fat-free mayonnaise

1 lime, juiced

1/2 teaspoon garlic powder

pinch of ground black pepper

Servings	9 (2 tablespoons per serving)
Prep Time	2 – 3 mins

PER SERVING

Calories	20
Protein	1 gram
Carbohydrates	4 grams
Fat	0 grams

> Place all of your ingredients in a medium-sized mixing bowl, mix well, and serve.

DESSERTS

Don't worry—I haven't forgotten the sweets. Don't think of your hard training as a license to indulge in treats regularly, though. You can kill your fat loss pretty quickly by simply adding a couple hundred calories too many each day.

That being said, there's nothing wrong with having a dessert every week or two. When I'm eating to gain muscle, I usually have one dessert per week (although some weeks I skip it—I'm not really into sugar). When I'm dieting to lose weight, I never have more than one small, (100-calorie) dessert per week, and I usually have one every two weeks.

The recipes I give here are better than your average dessert recipes in that they have no sugar and little fat. They use higher-quality carbs than your average junk at the store, and they are high in protein.

PROTEIN PUDDING

1 package sugar-free fat-free pudding

2 cups skim milk

2 scoops chocolate or vanilla whey protein powder (use same flavor as pudding)

Servings	2
Prep Time	Under 5 mins
Cooking Time	20 mins
PER SERVING	
Calories	266
Protein	32 grams
Carbohydrates	31 grams
Fat	1 gram

> Place all of your ingredients in a medium-sized bowl, stir together to combine everything, then mix with an electric hand mixer until it starts to thicken. Place in the refrigerator for at least 20 minutes to set.

PEACH COBBLER

Servings	6
Prep Time	10 – 15 mins
Cooking Time	30 – 35 mins

PER SERVING

Calories	154
Protein	11 grams
Carbohydrates	25 grams
Fat	1 gram

3 tablespoons blueberry, raspberry, strawberry, or mixed-fruit preserves

1 can (15 ounces) diced peaches in water or 100% juice, drained

1/2 cup low-fat cottage cheese

1/2 cup water

2 scoops vanilla whey protein powder

1/4 cup all-purpose flour

2 packets (2 grams) stevia or other sugar alternative

1/2 cup quick cooking oats

1 tablespoon honey

> Preheat the oven to 350°F.

> Pour the fruit preserves into an 8 x 8 inch baking dish and spread evenly. Add the peaches, spread evenly.

> In a mixing bowl, add the cottage cheese, water, protein powder, flour, and stevia. Mix well and pour over the peaches, spreading evenly.

> In a small mixing bowl, mix together the oats and honey. Pour over the cheese mixture.

> Bake for 30 minutes, let sit 20 minutes before serving.

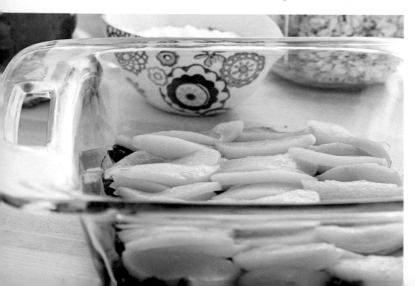

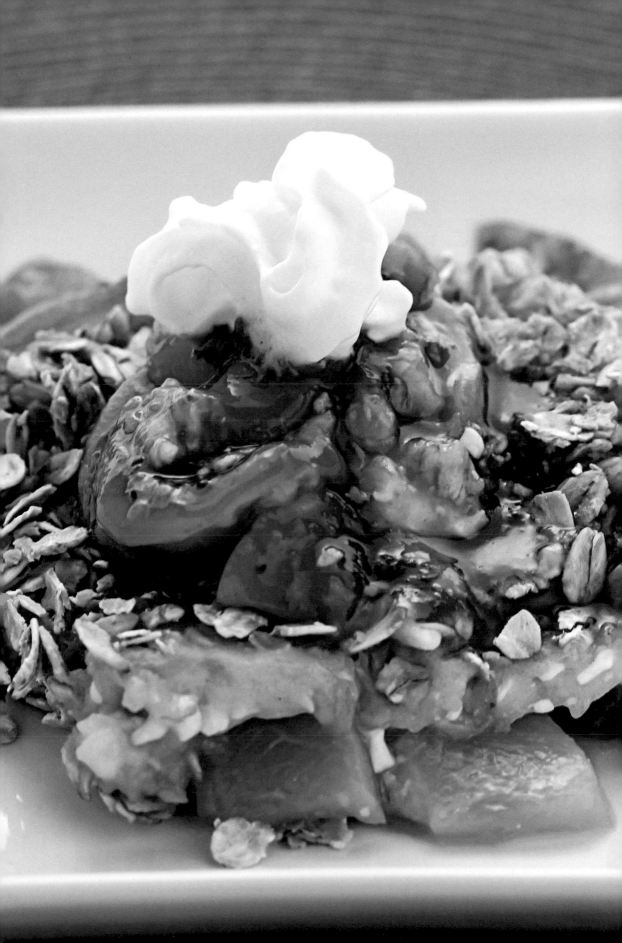

KEY LIME PIE

Servings	6
Prep Time	10 – 15 mins
Cooking Time	55 mins – 1 hr

PER SERVING

Calories	317
Protein	9 grams
Carbohydrates	61 grams
Fat	3 grams

4 sheets low-fat honey graham crackers, crushed into crumbs

1/2 cup applesauce

1 cup quick cooking oats

1 teaspoon ground cinnamon

3 egg yolks

1 can (14 ounces) fat-free condensed milk

1/3 cup key lime juice

2 cups fat-free frozen whipped topping, thawed

> Preheat the oven to 350°F.

> In a large mixing bowl, add the cracker crumbs, applesauce, oats, and cinnamon. Mix well. Remove 1 tablespoon of the mixture and set aside.

> Pour the cracker mixture in a 9 x 1.5 inch pie pan. Spread evenly and lightly pack it into and along the sides of the pan to form the crust. Bake for 15 minutes.

> In a medium-sized bowl, add the egg yolks, condensed milk, and key lime juice. Whisk until smooth. Reduce the oven temperature to 250°F, pour the juice mixture into the crust. Bake for 40 minutes, or until the filling is firm.

> Remove from heat, let sit until completely cool. Transfer to refrigerator for 4 – 6 hours, or until fully chilled. Top with a 2-inch layer of the whipped topping, sprinkle with the 1 tablespoon of crumb mixture, and serve.

PROTEIN MILKSHAKE

Servings	1
Prep Time	Under 5 mins

PER SERVING

Calories	259
Protein	25 grams
Carbohydrates	33 grams
Fat	2 grams

1 cup skim milk

1/2 cup low-fat frozen yogurt

1/2 teaspoon vanilla extract

1/2 scoop whey protein powder (your choice of flavor)

> Place all ingredients in a blender and blend on low for a few minutes, until desired consistency.

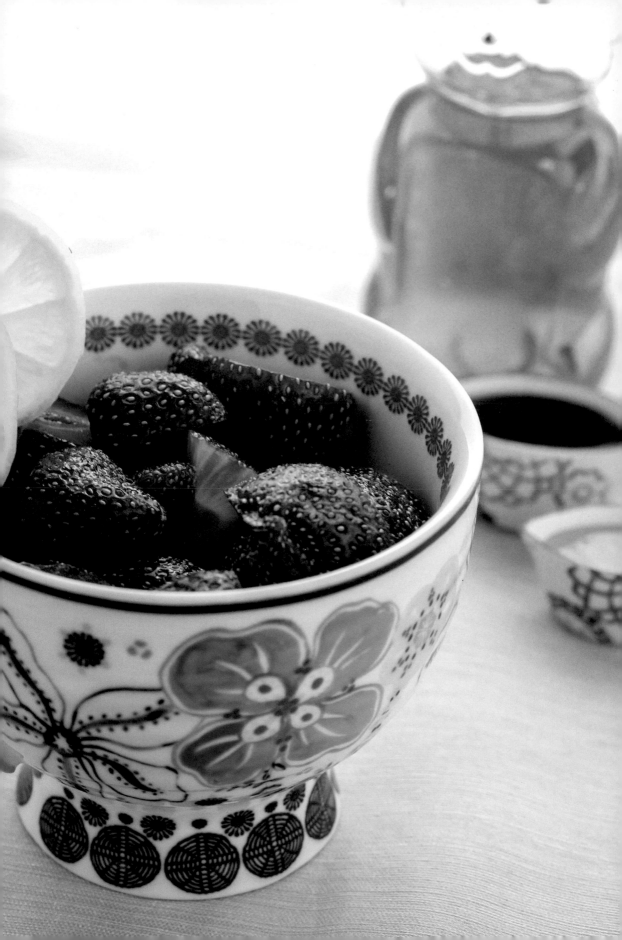

HONEY-BALSAMIC STRAWBERRIES

Servings	4
Prep Time	5 mins
PER SERVING	
Calories	117
Protein	2 grams
Carbohydrates	29 grams
Fat	1 gram

8 cups strawberries, washed, tops cut off, and halved

4 lemons, juiced

1 tablespoon balsamic vinegar

1 teaspoon honey

> In a large mixing bowl, add the strawberries and lemon juice, mix well and refrigerate for 2 hours.

> After the strawberries have chilled, in a separate bowl, mix the vinegar and honey. Drizzle the honey vinegar over the strawberries and serve.

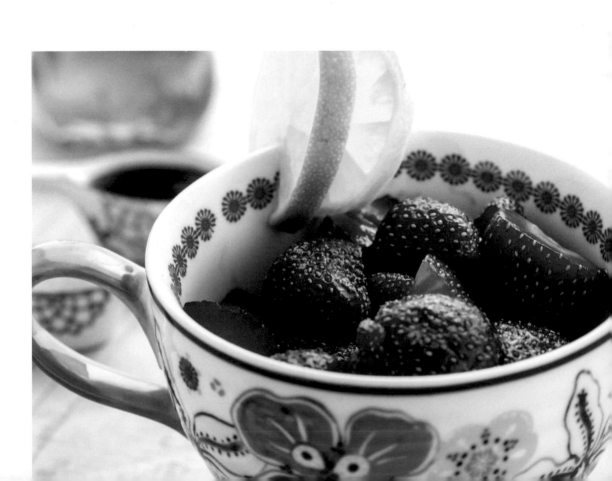

BONUS SPREADSHEET

First, I want to say THANK YOU for reading my book, *The Shredded Chef*.

I'm thrilled at how many people have written me to say how much they like the recipes for helping with losing weight, building muscle, and staying healthy.

Chances are you'd like to use the recipes in this book to plan out your daily meals. This handy spreadsheet will help!

In it you'll find a list of every recipe in the book along with their calories, protein, carbs, and fats. When you're planning your meals, all you have to do is skim over the spreadsheet and pick foods that fit your caloric and macronutritional targets. No need to browse through the entire cookbook!

Visit the link below to download this free spreadsheet today!

Visit WWW.BIT.LY/TSC-SPREADSHEET to get this spreadsheet now!

WOULD YOU DO ME A FAVOR?

Thank you for buying my book. I hope that you enjoy the recipes I've included and that they help you in your muscle-building and fat-torching endeavors.

I have a small favor to ask. Would you mind taking a minute to write a blurb on Amazon about this book? I check all my reviews and love to get feedback (that's the real pay for my work—knowing that I'm helping people).

Visit the following URL to leave me a review:

WWW.AMZN.TO/TSC-REVIEW

Also, if you have any friends or family that might enjoy this book, spread the love and lend it to them!

Now, I don't just want to sell you a book—I want to see you use what you've learned to build the body of your dreams.

As you work toward your goals, however, you'll probably have questions or run into some difficulties. I'd like to be able to help you with these, so let's connect up! I don't charge for the help, of course, and I answer questions from readers every day.

Here's how we can connect:

Facebook: facebook.com/muscleforlifefitness

Twitter: @muscleforlife

G+: gplus.to/MuscleForLife

And last but not least, my website is www.muscleforlife.com and if you want to write me, my email address is mike@muscleforlife.com.

Thanks again and I wish you the best!

Mike

ALSO BY MICHAEL MATTHEWS

Eat Green Get Lean: 100 Vegetarian and Vegan Recipes for Building Muscle, Getting Lean, and Staying Healthy

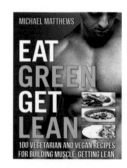

If you want to know how to build muscle and burn fat by eating delicious vegetarian and vegan meals that are easy to cook and easy on your wallet, then you want to read this book.

Visit www.muscleforlife.com to get this book!

Thinner Leaner Stronger: The Simple Science of Building the Ultimate Female Body

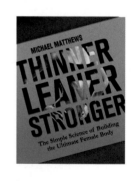

If you want to be toned, lean, and strong as quickly as possible without crash dieting, "good genetics," or wasting ridiculous amounts of time in the gym and money on supplements...regardless of your age...then you want to read this book.

Visit www.muscleforlife.com to get this book!

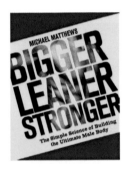

Bigger Leaner Stronger: The Simple Science of Building the Ultimate Male Body

If you want to be muscular, lean, and strong as quickly as possible, without steroids, good genetics, or wasting ridiculous amounts of time in the gym, and money on supplements...then you want to read this book.

Visit www.muscleforlife.com to get this book!

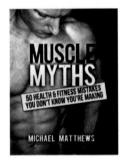

Muscle Myths: 50 Health & Fitness Mistakes You Don't Know You're Making

If you've ever felt lost in the sea of contradictory training and diet advice out there and you just want to know once and for all what works and what doesn't—what's scientifically true and what's false—when it comes to building muscle and getting ripped, then you need to read this book.

Visit www.muscleforlife.com to get this book!

Cardio Sucks! The Simple Science of Burning Fat Fast and Getting in Shape

If you're short on time and sick of the same old boring cardio routine and want to kick your fat loss into high gear by working out less and…heaven forbid…actually have some fun…then you want to read this new book.

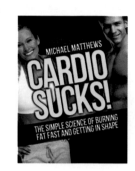

Visit www.muscleforlife.com to get this book!

Awakening Your Inner Genius

If you'd like to know what some of history's greatest thinkers and achievers can teach you about awakening your inner genius, and how to find, follow, and fulfill your journey to greatness, then you want to read this book today.

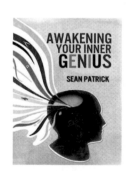

(I'm using a pen name for this book, as well as for a few other projects not related to health and fitness, but I thought you might enjoy it so I'm including it here.)

Visit www.yourinnergenius.com to get this book!